*Selected Papers of the
Commission on*

**Education
For Health
Administration
Volume II**

Selected Papers of the Commission on

EDUCATION FOR HEALTH ADMINISTRATION VOLUME II

Health Administration Press
Ann Arbor, 1975

Copyright © 1975 by The University of Michigan
Printed in the United States of America
Library of Congress Catalog Card No. 74-17537
ISBN No. 0-914904-05-1

*Published for the Commission on
Education in Health Administration
with the support of the W. K. Kellogg
Foundation*

Health Administration Press
M2240 School of Public Health
The University of Michigan
Ann Arbor, MI 48104
(313) 764-1380

The Commission on Education for Health Administration

James P. Dixon, Chairman
President, Antioch College

Robert A. Aldrich
*Vice President for Health Affairs
University of Colorado*

Manuel A. Bobenrieth
*Regional Advisor in Medical Care
  Administration Education,
Pan American Health Organization
World Health Organization*

Jacob Clayman
*Administrative Director
Industrial Union Department
AFL-CIO*

Lloyd F. Detwiller
*Administrator
Health Sciences Centre
University of British Columbia*

Amitai Etzioni
*Professor of Sociology
Columbia University
Director,
Center for Policy Research*

Joanne E. Finley
*State of New Jersey
Commissioner of Health*

David H. Gustafson
*Associate Professor
Industrial Engineering &
  Preventive Medicine
University of Wisconsin*

Lawrence A. Hill
*Vice President
American Hospital Association*

T.P. Hipkens
*Consultant
Appalachian Regional Hospitals, Inc.-
  Lexington, Kentucky*

Charles C. Johnson, Jr.
*Resident Manager
Malcolm Pirnie, Inc.
Consulting Environmental Engineers*

Joseph B. Mann
*Senior Vice President — Operations
New York City Health &
  Hospitals Corporation*

Grace Olivarez
*Director
Institute for Social Research &
  Development
Professor of Law
University of New Mexico*

Richard N. Rossett
*Professor of Economics and
  Preventive Medicine &
  Community Health
University of Rochester*

Reuel A. Stallones
*Dean, School of Public Health
University of Texas*

Karl D. Yordy
*Senior Program Officer
Institute of Medicine
National Academy of Sciences*

Panel of Educational Consultants

Paul B. Corneley
*Consultant to the Executive
 Medical Officer,
United Mine Workers of America
 Welfare and Retirement Fund*

Gary L. Filerman
*Executive Director
Association of University
 Programs in Health
 Administration*

William N. Hubbard, Jr.
President, The Upjohn Company

Jerry W. Miller
*Director, Office on Educational Credit
American Council on Education*

Eugene Feingold
*Chairman
Department of Medical
 Care Organization
The University of Michigan*

Theodore Heimarck
*Director
Program in Hospital Administration
Concordia College*

Carl A. Meilecke
*Director, Division of
 Health Services Administration
University of Alberta*

Stephen B. Plumer
*Educational Consultant
Potomac, Maryland*

Commission Staff

Charles J. Austin
Study Director

*On Leave During The Study From Xavier University Graduate
Program in Hospital and Health Administration. Presently Dean
of Graduate Studies, Trinity University, San Antonio.*

Janet A. Strauss
Assistant Study Director

Éva K. Winters
Secretary

Contents

Foreword ix
  by Karl Yordy

Preface xi

I. **Reports of Special Projects Conducted by Commission Members**

  Accountability in Health Administration 3
    by Amitai Etzioni

  Roles and Training for Future Health Systems Engineers 25
    by David H. Gustafson, Glenwood L. Rowse, and Nancy J. Howes

  The Demand for Hospital Administrators 61
    by Roger Feldman and Richard N. Rossett

II. **Report of Commission Research**

  Education for Health Administration: A Statistical Profile 71
    by Charles J. Austin, Daniel A. Clark, and James A. Ball

III. **Report of a Field Research Study**

  The Role of the Health Services Administrator and Implications for Education 147
    by Robert F. Allison, William L. Dowling, and Fred C. Munson

IV. **Papers Presented at the Institute on New Approaches to Education for Health Administration**

  Public Accountability and Human Services Orientation in Health Administration 185
    by Fred E. Mondragon

  Putting Health into Health Administration 198
    by George A. Lamb and Julius B. Richmond

  Generic Versus Specialist Aspects of Health Administration 213
    by William C. Richardson

The Future Health Administrators as Viewed by Others 229
by Nathan J. Stark

Credentialing for Health Administration 257
by Jerry W. Miller

Career Mobility and Lifelong Learning in Health Administration 275
by Stephen B. Plumer

Health Administration Issues: Implications for Education of Administrators 298
by James R. Kimmey

The Organizational Network of Education for Health Administration 317
by David B. Starkweather

Foreword

Early in the Commission's deliberations it became clear that a wide variety of data, information and opinion should be brought to bear on the issues to be considered. We sought to meet this need in a variety of ways.

Commission members with particular interests and expertise undertook special projects concerning public accountability in health administration; the use of specialists, such as systems engineers, to greatest advantage in health administration practice; and the probable demand for certain kinds of health administrators. Other research efforts, undertaken by the Commission Study Director and by a group at the University of Michigan School of Public Health under an HEW-HSMHA contract, concerned the nature of existing health administration educational efforts and the nature of day-to-day health administration practice.

To broaden the bases for Commission conclusions still further, an Institute on New Approaches to Education for Health Administration, supported by the W. K. Kellogg Foundation, was planned around a number of issues germane to both education and practice. The eight papers prepared for discussion at the Institute brought other considerations and points of view to bear on Commission concerns.

These reports and discussion papers represent analytical research, information from surveys of fact and opinion, and speculation about possibilities for change in the education of health administrators. All of this material, though not all in its final report form, was available to the almost one hundred people who attended the Institute in New Orleans in January, 1974, which I had the pleasure of chairing.

For two-and-one-half days the eight areas of concern addressed in the discussion papers were investigated, primarily in small discussion groups of carefully chosen participants. The plenary sessions gave opportunity for refocusing and development of consensus on the issues facing the Commission, and for the Commission to define prudent boundaries for its conclusions and recommendations.

All of the work and ideas reported and described in this volume was considered by the Commission and influenced our recommendations. We are grateful for the help and support of all those who participated in the Institute.

                                    Karl D. Yordy
                                    Chairman, Institute on
                                          New Approaches to
                                          Education for Health
                                          Administration
                                    Washington, D.C.
                                    October 17, 1974

Preface

This second volume of the Commission's report contains papers generated to supplement other Commission efforts, in areas that seemed to need special attention, and in which special expertise was available.

The first three papers are reports on research projects undertaken by Commission members in fields of their special interest and knowledge: public accountability, use of specialists in health administration practice, and supply and demand for administrative personnel.

To provide a different sort of data, five questionnaire surveys were undertaken, under supervision of the Commission's Study Director. These sought information on existing graduate and undergraduate health administration education programs, and on how graduate students, graduate program graduates, and employers of those graduates, view current and needed educational offerings. Collection and analysis of the survey data were carried out over much of the Commission's life and provided bases for major conclusions and recommendations. All five surveys are reported in the paper by Austin, Ball, and Clark.

A problem central to all of the Commission's deliberations was identification and interpretation of practicing administrators' roles and day-to-day responsibilities. The Allison-Dowling-Munson paper in this volume reports on a preliminary inquiry into these matters and supplements Austin's working paper on the definition of health administration, included in the first volume of this report. As is indicated, the work reported by Allison et al. was supported by a DHEW-HSMHA contract.

To further enhance both the quantity and quality of information at the Commission's disposal, the W. K. Kellogg Foundation additionally supported an Institute on New Approaches to Education for Health Administration, held in New Orleans in January 1974. As bases for discussions by groups of invited participants, eight papers were contracted for and submitted to the Commission, covering as many aspects of health administration education and practice. Building on the contents of Commission working and survey papers, the Institute papers which comprise the final section of this volume lent further perspective to the Commission's work and stimulated thoughtful contributions by those invited to attend the Institute.

Inevitably, differences of approach and suggested solution are reflected in the papers published here. Such diversity was viewed by the Commission as both constructive and thought-provoking. We express our particular appreciation to those who researched and wrote these papers, and who thereby made substantial contributions to the results of our study.

                                              James P. Dixon
                                              Chairman
                                              October 17, 1974

Part I

Reports of Special
Projects Conducted by
Commission Members

Authors in Part I

Amitai Etzioni, Ph.D.
Director, Center for Policy Research
(Professor of Sociology, Columbia University)

Roger Feldman
Economist, Economic Analysis Branch
Department of Health, Education and Welfare

David H. Gustafson, Ph.D.
Associate Professor
Industrial Engineering and Preventive Medicine
University of Wisconsin

Nancy J. Howes, Ph.D.
Assistant Professor
Education Administration
State University of New York at Albany

Richard N. Rossett, Ph.D.
Chairman, Department of Economics
University of Rochester

Glenwood L. Rowse, M.S., Industrial Engineering
  and Curriculum and Instruction
Research Specialist
University of Wisconsin

Accountability in Health Administration*

Alternative Conceptions of Accountability

Preface

We shall first discuss alternative conceptions of accountability in health administration, then the consequences of this analysis for the education of health administrators. The separation is doubly necessary as: (1) we must have an understanding of the underlying forces before we can formulate a sound educational policy; and (2) an analysis such as the one which follows is in itself a major potential educational tool. It can serve in the important task of sensitizing health administrators to contrasting conceptions of accountability.

The Symbolic Uses of Accountability

Speakers and writers calling for greater accountability typically employ the term in three concrete contexts: to refer to greater responsibility and responsiveness to the needs of patients; to allude to greater attention to the community (generally a euphemism for blacks, Mexican-Americans, American Indians or other minorities, especially a large minority living in the vicinity of the hospital); or to greater commitment to values (e.g., as in the phrase "higher standards of morality"). The unifying thread is the symbolic use of the term account-

---

* by Amitai Etzioni, Ph.D. This is a preliminary report of a much more encompassing project undertaken for the Commission on Education for Health Administration with the support of the W. K. Kellogg Foundation. The project was undertaken by Amitai Etzioni with Harry Greenfield. Pamela Doty and Nancy Castleman served as research assistants for this part of the report. The author is grateful to Charles Austin for comments on a previous draft.

ability. Though it may not necessarily be—indeed perhaps rarely is—the consciously intended meaning, the chief definition of this term which, in fact, emerges is that of "accountability as gesture." The hallmark of accountability as gesture is that it is pure norm with little or no instrumentality attached. That is, the speaker or writer advocating accountability fails to follow up the use of the term by outlining specific arrangements, e.g., that patients be made the controlling force on hospital boards or that minorities be allotted a third of the beds, etc.; or, if such suggestions are made at all, the virtue held out for them is fully matched by their vagueness.

Making "more information" available to the public is an example of such a suggestion, as in the following quotation from a statement of policy and program by the Community Health Institute (New York City): "Those who provide health services to the public must be accountable to that public. This then requires that the people have access to all the relevant information needed to make accountability real. Accountability to the public is essential for public control."[1] Thus the prime function of "accountability" here is that by using the word the speaker declares himself "on the side of the angels." Rather than outlining a mechanism he is articulating or reaffirming a value position.

The sociological significance of such expressions, gestures, and utterances, however, is more varied than one might immediately think. The point can be readily illustrated by reflecting on the differential significance of the word "integration" as used in the early sixties, in each case symbolically, by the following types of persons: a white legislator endorsing integration to his black constituents, but failing to introduce or support bills enforcing specific aspects of integration; a black civil rights leader such as Martin Luther King or Roy Wilkins building a social movement; a white minister exhorting his white congregation in Scarsdale against racism.

The first use is inauthentic and manipulative. When divorced from any systematic efforts to promote actual attainment of the desired values, accountability becomes a thin cover for inaction, a Sunday only value mechanically acknowledged in a secular form of lip service. This kind of accountability can be easily and vociferously endorsed by boards of trustees, insurance lobbyists, and others in positions of power whose recitations of the phrase serve as a substitute for actual accountability. It becomes then only a verbal concession, like the rhetoric of the Kerner Commission Report, with little provision for follow-through, as a direct drain of the pressures to do something about the situation.

Murray Edelman, in his book, *The Symbolic Uses of Politics,* devoted a good deal of space to a discussion of such hortatory uses of political slogans. According to Edelman, there is the solemn ritual incantation of political slogans by those in charge of formulating or carrying out policy that is unaccompanied by any effective attempts to achieve the goals incanted. This is particularly likely to occur in a situation where a large but politically unorganized group which feels itself threatened, desires certain resources or power. Opposed to the fulfillment of their wishes is a small, politically organized group or groups with an effective interest in the resources or the substantive power claimed.[2] Under such circumstances, it is tempting for the politicians or administrators to satisfy the desires of those in the first groups through symbolic reassurance that they are not being ignored or that their interests will be protected. Often, symbolic reassurance from power-wielders will provoke quiescence in an unorganized group—at the very least because it takes the edge off dissatisfaction and makes the difficulties of mobilization greater.[3] This quiescence may be quite temporary, soon yielding to a reawakening of demand and a resentment over being manipulated. But those who merely mouth accountability do not concern themselves with the longer run. In this vein Wilbur Rich has written in *Administration in Mental Health* that:

> Mental health administrators . . . view mandates from politicians for accountability as a political games posture that will relax itself after the budget hearings. Administrators affect a defensive posture and tighten their monitoring of operating facilities to discourage public incidents. Curious legislators have to be 'educated' and administrators need to be told they are not running a private domain. The media report these encounters as public officials overseeing the bureaucracy. This reaction has almost become an annual game in which each participant is aware of the rules, and the public is led to believe something is being done. After the usefulness of the game has been exhausted, everybody agrees that a better job needs to be done and goes home (Edelman 1967). However, the scarcity of public resources and the coming of the 'true believer'—the researcher— have made the game more difficult to play.[4]

Following the analogy made to the word "integration" which was mentioned earlier, political and social movement leaders also use slogans and cue-words in their attempts to mobilize followers. Perhaps they even use the same word that is being used by the power wielders in an attempt to provide symbolic reassurance to potential followers. In this context, however, though the use is still symbolic, the meaning is quite different. While group leaders may still be dealing largely with gestures rather than mechanisms, accountability in this instance serves as a rallying point around which mobilization can be affected and a movement built. In such a situation the demand for accountability becomes a shared symbol of all those individuals galvanized into a political force which aims at seeking and gaining specific concessions.[5] Once there is such an organized force, the question of how accountability can be actualized may be: confronted immediately; only a step away; or deliberately deferred as a bargaining technique.

Somewhere in between the "coopting" inauthentic use of slogans as political tranquilizers unresponsive to basic needs and the issue-flagging, group-rallying use by leaders seeking to mobilize a constituency, is the use of "accountability" as the banner of a campaign for moral education. Typically such a campaign is undertaken by one professional vis à vis his fellows or by a concerned but unself-interested outsider. The moral educator views those proselytized in a manner very much akin to the way a socially conscious minister views his congregation: as persons who are basically anxious to do right by their values and their fellows but whose behavior is not what it should be either because of lack of knowledge and having been improperly taught or because they have not been reminded of their duties or because insufficiently "good" models suitable for emulation have been set before them. Thus, exhortation, moral suasion, lay preaching, example setting are relied upon instead of introducing new accountability mechanisms —not to be inauthentic but because these approaches are sincerely believed to be effective.

Dr. Avedis Donabedian attributes the tendency in health administration to emphasize moral education over regulation to the norm of colleaguality among physicians and the weakness of the formal and informal controls administrators have vis à vis physicians. He writes,

> The administrator must . . . determine the proper balance between the educational objectives of quality assessment and the need to deter and detect careless or incompetent practice. . . .
> In real life, the answer appears to depend in part on the role and influence of the practicing physicians on the program. Wherever this influence is small, as in some health insurance programs, there is either no responsibility for quality or, at best, emphasis is placed on the identification and correction of abuse that border on the criminal. Wherever the role of the practicing physician is significantly large or dominant, the emphasis may fall so predominantly on the educational objective that the disciplinary objective is in danger of being ignored or explicitly excluded.[6]

Dr. Donabedian goes on to explain the reasons for this imbalance:

> Fundamentally, the control of behavior within the medical profession is brought about not by the coercive power of superior authority, but by the

operation of ethical standards that prescribe responsibility to patients and sensitivity to the good opinion of colleagues. This fundamental orientation is reinforced by notions concerning the nature and frequency of deviations from accepted practice and what accounts for them. It is asserted that most physicians are motivated to provide good care and to use the hospital in an appropriate manner. Deviations are believed to be caused by occasional inattention, by gradual, unintentional drift into bad habits or technical obsolescence, or by pervasive administrative and organizational constraints over which the physician has little control. Flagrant abuse is said to be a rare phenomenon. As a consequence, significant improvements in the levels of care, and savings in hospital days inappropriately used, are not likely to be achieved by detecting and correcting abuse, but by bringing about smaller, and more pervasive, changes in the practice of a much larger number of physicians. It is the cumulative effect of these smaller adjustments, influencing the mass of physicians, that is expected to pay the greatest dividends. Finally, any approach that leads to the exclusion or elimination of specified physicians from program participation is considered to be socially undesirable because it simply permits the physician to continue practice in the general community, unsupported and unsupervised. . . .[7]

As different as the different uses of the term "accountability" that have been discussed so far are, however, they all rely upon it as a symbol rather than as a social force and, unfortunately, tend to run into one another. As a result, on many occasions, when health administrators talk favorably about accountability, one has a difficult time discerning whether their gestures are inauthentic, rallying, or educationalistic. Moreover, their social consequences will depend in part on the other accountability processes, which are explored next.

Accountability as *Realpolitik*

A contrasting view of accountablity of health administrators is that of an existing pattern of administration and government which reflects at any particular point in time the sum total of the forces working on the health system, those working to maintain the status quo, and those seeking to reshape it. Such an outlook adapts the interest group theories of politics espoused by such political analysts as Robert Dahl, David Truman, V. O. Key and Earl Latham.[8] From this perspective, the hospital is viewed as a polity, affected by its members and by outside forces, in the continual act of restructuring. Apart from its bookkeeping and managerial functions in the narrow sense, hospital administration is seen as a political process through which various groupings negotiate, confront, or adjust their claims. Thus, accountability becomes the actual degree to which the hospital administration is responsive to the claims and demands of the particular interests of doctors, nurses, union, activist patients, etc.

The hospital administrator is seen as being located at the center of this process—the focal point of the pressure—not at the top, in charge. The hospital administrator's position in this theory in fact is analagous to that of a billard ball in a physics diagram upon which various forces impinge. Typically, the hospital administrator's actions are seen as almost totally determined by various partisan interest group pressures; predicting the behavior of the administrator then is a matter of knowing the coefficients of strength of the various groups.

Even when hospital administrators are seen as having views of their own and a modicum of autonomy, they are not seen as representing the interests of the polity as a whole—but of having their own vested interests, which are similarly parochial to those of the other pressure groups. In general, the interests imputed to administrators are those of the bureaucrat seeking either to expand his domain and, most especially, to defend his own incumbency in authority.[9] Such a view of hospital administration and accountability we label as *Realpolitik* because it is characterized by the fact that power is viewed as the only significant variable.

The rules of *Realpolitik* are fairly well known. To list them here, briefly, is of course, to report and not to bless their existence. By and large, groups with more status, income, and education have more power and hence make the system relatively more accountable to them. That is, they have more leverage. Accordingly, one would expect a typical American voluntary hospital (and its administration and administrator) to be most accountable to the physicians and/or trustees, less so to the nurses and aides, least so to the patients, and especially inattentive to the poor, uneducated, non-paying customers. In terms of the typical American community, one would expect the hospital to be most responsive to the local business community, and less so to other groups. As a rule, following *Realpolitik* we would expect more responsiveness to government agencies of various levels, less to consumer groups and advocates.

Different types of hospitals—municipal, proprietary, voluntary, etc.—are expected to vary in the groups they respond to most readily and in the kinds of power base which has the greatest leverage. For instance we might expect voluntary hospitals to be rather more insulated from the pressures of city politics than the municipal hospitals but rather more dependent upon the good will and continued munificence of the cities' first families.[10]

Some evidence that different interest groups possess differential amounts of power in different types of hospitals is given by an analysis of data collected by the Michigan Health and Social Security Institute on the membership of the boards of trustees of forty-eight Detroit area hospitals. They found that in the category of not-for-profit hospitals which were neither osteopathic, governmental, or religiously run, more than 50 percent of the board members were executives and lawyers. By contrast, on boards of hospitals owned by local government, executives and lawyers numbered no more than 11 percent of the board members. On the local government-owned hospital boards in general, there was less business representation and greater community diversification, including public officials, educators, union officials, foremen, a consumer consultant, a safety consultant, a housewife, a farmer, and an industrial relations consultant.[11]

According to a *Realpolitik* analysis, groups will also differ in their leverage over time, depending on the extent to which they are organized and mobilized to affect the particular polity under consideration. Thus, if the physicians act chiefly as individuals, they will obtain fewer resources than if they set up hospital-wide committees, aiming to insure that their collective preference will carry the day. And, as a rule, unionized hospital workers will be more accounted to than unorganized ones. Even patients, represented by patients' advocates, ombudsmen, lawyers, or consumer representatives—being weak and easy to deflect—will, according to this view, gain in more ways than they would without any of these organizations and mobilizing devices.

Empirical support for the view that the nature of the power constellations in hospitals changes over time is given by Charles Perrow in an historical case study tracing changes in goals and power in a voluntary hospital from 1885 to 1958.[12] The period 1885 to 1929 was found to be one of trustee domination, reflecting the overriding importance of obtaining capital and community legitimation. The significantly weaker power of the doctors testified to the still primitive state of medical science at the time. The hospital was organized as a charity hospital under Jewish auspices and its prime function was to provide free care to impoverished Jews and other needy persons. From 1929 to 1942 the balance of power shifted to the doctors, a change directly related to the enormous technical advances made in medical science beginning in the first 30 years of the century and continuing on. The emphasis on free care declined greatly and, in line with the priorities of the doctors, service was oriented toward paying patients. And the hospital began to seek prestige in terms that the medical profession recognized: through research. From 1942 to 1952, an administrative challenge arose to correct some of the abuse that had arisen due to medical domination. Because the administrator was a doctor, he could achieve hegemony in the medical area as well as the strictly administrative aspects of the hospital. The period of multiple leadership (1952–1958) began when a new administrator was hired and a clear demarcation made between the expressive and instrumental elites, giving each increased autonomy in his own area.

Meanwhile, a conflict between the previous administrator and the medical staff had led the former to seek allies amongst the hitherto dormant trustees. A temporary coalition was formed between the administrator and the reactivated trustees but eventually the board evolved into an independent third force. By 1958 then the leadership included three roughly equal parties: the administration, the trustees and the doctors. Multiple leadership according to Perrow leads to three types of decision-making—the fortuitous convergence of interests, segregated decision-making and the piecemeal accumulation of small victories. Though the dominance of one group is avoided, the balance of power places a premium on harmony and avoidance of conflict with the drawback that long range planning tends to be neglected since it could expose conflicting interests.[13]

This hard-headed view suggests that the phrase "more accountable" is meaningless; the question is: to whom? The implication is that accountability to one group means almost by definition, less accountability to another. Implicit in the *Realpolitik* position is that values per se—e.g., as represented by the normal education of the administrator—count for almost nil. A change in the relative power of the various groups is the only factor which could be expected to produce a significant change in accountability.

THE FORMAL, LEGAL APPROACH

Many in the health field subscribe to a view of accountability which defines it in legal or formal terms. The emphasis is on instituting "checks and balances." In the academic world, such an approach was once current in political science. While it has lost in following over the past twenty years, it is still quite popular in the field of public administration. Game theory and cybernetics are chiefly in this vein of thinking.

In hospital administration, this approach sees the administrator as having to be made "accountable" to one or more authorities—the board, his superior, the law, etc. and much ink is shed to clarify these legalities.

A case point is the question: if a doctor misbehaves in a hospital, who is legally accountable, the doctor alone, the hospital and its administrator alone or both?

In a recent California malpractice case, Albert Gonzales vs. John G. Nork, M.D. and Mercy General Hospital of Sacramento, the judge found both the hospital and the doctor responsible for the patient's damages.[14] He awarded Gonzales $1.7 million in compensatory damages against both defendants and $2 million in punitive damages against the physician alone. The hospital attorneys had argued that since the medical staff of the hospital was self-governing with regard to professional work, the hospital could not be held responsible for Nork's performance of needless surgery on Gonzales and on others, most of whom suffered neurologic deficits as a result. The judge disagreed stating, "The hospital, by virtue of its custody of the patient, owes him a duty of care; this duty includes the obligation to protect him from acts of malpractice by his independently retained physician who is a member of the hospital staff if the hospital knows or has reason to know or should have known that such acts were likely to occur.[15] He then ruled that the repeated "bad" surgical results obtained by Dr. Nork should have been recognized by Mercy's peer review committees, set up pursuant to the hospital's bylaws, and that Dr. Nork's surgical practice should have been restricted.

Similar rulings were handed down in a number of other recent cases: a 1965 Illinois Supreme Court decision, Darling vs. Charleston Community Memorial Hospital, a 1972 Nevada Supreme Court decision, George L. Moore vs. the Board of Carson Tahoe Hospital, and a 1972 Arizona Appelate decision, Kay L. Purcell vs. Zimbleman.[16]

Along related lines, there have been attempts to make hospitals more accountable to the public-at-large by requiring them to file detailed financial statements and various mechanisms have been proposed to make such financial statements easily accessible to interested parties. In addition, laws have been put through requiring the participation of consumers on Hill-Burton advisory councils and in state and regional Comprehensive Health Planning organizations.[17]

Recent changes in hospital accreditation procedures are permitting consumers and consumer organizations to participate in the accreditation process. Citizens do this by learning when the biannual accreditations surveys of hospitals in their areas are to be held and by being present at an information interview to state complaints as they relate to the standards of the Joint Commission on Accreditation of Hospitals.[18]

And in an effort to make doctors and hospitals more accountable to the government in the spending of Medicare and Medicaid monies, Congress recently enacted the PSRO legislation designed to subject old and poor patients' admission to a hospital to pre-admission review in all but emergency cases by local committees of doctors. A tougher proposal requiring an in-hospital committee review of Medicare admissions to crack down on needless hospitalization or protracted stays was dropped by the Social Security Administration after drawing heavy fire from the A.M.A.[19]

Structural changes within the hospital are similar measures, because they work on the basis of changes in formal definitions. Thus, requiring that hospitals have a consumer representative on the board is a case in point; it is said to make the hospital more accessible. Following this logic, the O.E.O. guidelines dictated that O.E.O. and other neighborhood health centers funded by the Public Health Service had to form either governing boards or advisory committees, composed of at least one-third "democratically selected representatives of the poor."[20]

Similarly there have been experiments in some health units with patients' advocates, patients' rights organizations and formalized grievance procedures. For example, at Yale-New Haven Hospital a patient's advocate program was set up by the Dixwell Legal Rights organization.[21] The woman hired to be the patients' advocate was a resident of the community, had thirteen years experience as a practical nurse and was given 10 months paralegal training by the Dixwell organization.

At Coler Hospital in New York, a chronic disease facility, three different patients' organizations whose stances range from conservative to radical change managed through union-style action to substantially increase the civil rights of the chronic care patients housed in the institution. Among the gains achieved: the city has been forced to register over 350 voters on Welfare Island, many of whom have been residents of the hospital for more than ten years, and voting machines have been promised for election day. In addition, the hospital's right to open mail before giving it to patients—particularly Social Security checks, which the hospital then distributed along with sign-over slips—has been challenged in court.

The Martin Luther King Center in the Bronx, New York, has set up a patients' rights program which includes a definition of patients' rights, mechanisms for dissemination of these rights to the community and the establishment of a systematic procedure for their enforcement. All registrants at the Center are to receive a patients' rights manual, a grievance form and information about the grievance procedure. The rights covered include: privacy, confidentiality and consent, all explained in concrete terms readily understandable to the registrants.[22]

Many social scientists are skeptical of such formal and legal accountability mechanisms. According to the most popular introductory textbook in sociology, *Sociology* by Leonard Broom and Philip Selznick:[23]

> The rules of the formal system account for much but by no means all of the patterned behavior in associations. The phrase 'informal structure' is used to denote those patterns that emerge from the spontaneous interaction of personalities and groups within the organization. . . . An organization's informal structure is made up of the patterns that develop when the participants face persistent problems that are not provided for by the formal system. These problems arise in a variety of ways:
>
> **1. Impersonality of the formal system.** The definite rules and prescribed rules of the formal structure are necessarily impersonal. . . . In practice, it is often necessary to reach individuals as *person*s, if their best efforts and their highest loyalty are to be mustered. . . .
>
> **2. Lag of the formal system** . . . the formal system of an organization tends to lag behind changes in its operations. . . . Despite the lag, those who do the work must solve new problems, even if these problems have not yet been recognized officially and there are no rules to meet them. . . . The temporary solution may be an informal consultation. . . .
>
> **3. Generality of the formal system.** The rules that make up the formal system are general. . . . In every organization there are some informal patterns that provide more detailed control than the formal system. In time some of these patterns may become formalized; others will remain outside official recognition. . . . By keeping rules general, ways of acting may be tested informally before they are given official approval. . . .
>
> **4. Personal problems and interests.** . . . Informal structure arises as the individual brings into play problems and interests other than those defined by his role in the organization.[24]

In the health care system, the consumer representative often turns out to be not the peoples' representative, but a businessman rather similar to the other board members in background and outlook. Or such positions may be monopolized by various types of "health professionals" who may not always agree with the doctors, but who are not average consumers either. In addition, consumers on hospital boards often learn that formal entitlements do not necessarily confer real power just as stockholders long ago discovered in business corporations. The power wielders may hold their own meeting in a backroom prior to the formal meeting which then becomes a mere ceremony. Or, the doctors and administrators may have their way via the phenomenon of partisan analysis—if the consumers have no independent source of information they may have no way of arriving at and documenting a point of view opposing the administrative one. Similarly, the aura of expertise surrounding doctors and administrators vs. the low social status of the consumer representatives can be expected to contribute to the likelihood that the consumer representatives defer to the hospital officials. In addition, while the doctors and administrators have a continuing personal vested interest in the affairs of the hospital, the motivations of consumer representatives are more likely to be altruistic. Unless the position of consumer representative is one which confers great prestige in the person's social circle, or there is some other reward, there seems little incentive to attend meetings often and regularly and to engage in the necessary self-education. It seems almost inevitable for enthusiasm to decline over time.[25]

There are analagous problems with relying on consumer grievance procedures to insure "accountability." The chief drawback is that consumers are usually quite unable to judge for themselves the technical aspects of the medical care they receive. The truth of this observation is strikingly highlighted by the results of a study in which judgments of expert assessors were compared with the opinions of those who received the care in question. "For cases in which care was judged to have been excellent or good, 86 percent of patients expressed the opinion that they had received the best care. For cases judged by experts to have been fair or poor, 75 percent of patients felt they had received the best care. At the same time, in the second category of cases only five percent of patients said the care received had been 'not good'."[26]

At first glance, the social science caveat, "not all that glitters with accountability truly enhances it," seems to be revalidated from data on the health system. Nevertheless, on balance, formal mechanisms do have an effect—especially when coupled with efforts to build consensus around values and to mobilize power through coalition building as discussed below. Thus, a study of the accomplishments of thirty-seven Massachusetts Mental Health and Retardation Area Boards on which citizen participation had been required by legislation revealed four separate types of board accomplishment. Each one resulted from a different strategy pursued by the board: service creation or improvement, mobilization of outside resources (from state and federal government), achievement of local autonomy (mobilization of resources from the private sector or the local government) and coordination (integration of the efforts of a variety of social agencies).[27]

Although consumer representation on decision-making and advisory bodies overseeing health units has received the most attention as the solution to the problems of instituting accountability to the public at large, it is by no means the only mechanism available. Another promising approach is that of the regularly scheduled Comprehensive Health Audit (CHA). The principle behind the notion of the Comprehensive Health Audit is essentially the same as that behind the annual financial audit in the corporate world. In the case of the corporate financial audit, the law requires that an outside expert licensed by the government (a C.P.A.) review the books of the joint stock company on a yearly basis so as to ensure accountability of the firm and its managers to the stockholders or legal owners of the corporation.

The Comprehensive Health Audit would entail a regular assessment of cost-consciousness and quality of care delivered in each hospital by an outside team of health auditors licensed by the government. The chief advantages of the Comprehensive Health Audit are that: (1) it accords well with the American philosophy of harnessing the profit motive in the service of the public interest; (2) it avoids the necessity of setting up a costly and cumbersome governmental regulatory apparatus (which as we know from historical experience has typically ended by serving the purposes of those it was intended to watchdog); and (3) it relies upon a tried and true mechanism, known to be efficient in one area and transfers it to a closely related field. The chief disadvantage of the Comprehensive Health Audit is that input measurements are so much more refined than output measures. Until more accurate output indices are developed, C.H.A.'s will have to employ fairly crude measures and their evaluations will not be nearly so reliable as the traditional financial audit.[28]

A Guidance Approach

The following view of accountability—the "guidance" approach—is, I should hasten to admit, the view closest to my heart. It took me six hundred odd-pages to spell it out elsewhere.[29] Here, I will simply suggest its chief points relevant to the issue at hand.

As I see it, accountability is based on a variety of inter-acting forces, not one lone attribute or mechanism. The direction health administrators take, in accountability as in other matters, is affected by all the factors already listed and some others still to be mentioned. In part, they respond to articulations of rights on the part of "the community," its leaders, the press, etc., that is, to claims of accountability. In part, their accountability is circumscribed and delineated by the legalities and formalities of the state, and so on. Hence, changes in any and all of these factors are effective ways to change the level and scope of accountability; none of them is all-inclusive.

Moreover, several missing elements must still be added to complete the analysis: for example, in contrast to those who see power as the core explanatory factor, I see accountability as having both a power and a moral base, in the sense that the values which administrators internalize (as well as those of other participants, both in the health unit under consideration and persons acting on it from the outside), do both affect the direction the health unit takes. Thus, in a recent study by the Center for Policy Research, Dr. Steven Beaver and Dr. Rosita Albert found (in a study of which I am the principal investigator, supported by NIMH) that the administrators of several hospitals studied were more progressive on several counts, than either the people in the area served by the hospital, or their patient-advocate, activist leaders.

For example, neighborhood residents, community leaders, and hospital administrators in a major United States city were asked:

> Which of these three kinds of health care do you think is the most important for this community? The three types are: A. Routine problems (checkups, maternal and child care, dental and eye care, ordinary sicknesses); B. Care of major body illnesses (heart problems, cancer, operations); C. Care for socially relevant problems (drug addiction, mental illness, alcoholism).

While a full 80 percent of the hospital administrators chose the socially relevant problems as the most important kind of health care problem for the neighborhood, smaller proportions of the neighborhood residents and community leaders choose this alternative, 60 and 52 percent respectively. Routine problems were judged as most important by 31 percent of the community residents, 35 percent of the leaders, and 20 percent of the hospital administrators. Major body illnesses were seen as the most important health care problem to 9 percent of the neighborhood dwellers, 14 percent of their leaders, and to none of the administrators. Thus, while majorities of all three groups believe that problems such as drug addiction, mental illness, and alcoholism are the major health problems of the community under study, a clearly higher percentage of the hospital administrators holds to this view. While the differences are not sizable, it is nevertheless significant that they remained consistent across a broad spectrum of questions answered by the three groups.

This study but illustrates what we all know from personal experience: administrators are not neutral beings. They have sentiments, preferences, and above all, values—although, of course, they differ greatly among themselves as to what they value, how clearly they perceive their values, and how far they are willing to go in promoting their values against those of others, say those of M.D.'s, if a difference should become evident. The content and intensity of these value commitments are in part affected by the administrator's education, a point to which we shall return.

The administrator need not be merely a broker of power, a meeting point of various internal and external pressures which he adapts the way a vectogram would; adapting to the strongest pressure at the moment, although in reality quite a few administrators act in this way. Aside from his personal values and position of authority in the structure, which give him a separate backbone, i.e., a measure of direction other than the *Realpolitik* of give and take, there is, in addition, an opportunity for creative leadership.

I do not see the capacity for leadership as consisting of abstract, moralistic character traits; I see these as specific skills. The object is not to fly in the face of reality or power groups, nor to wildly pursue Utopian notions of social justice or accountability—such an administrator is all too likely to be quickly expelled—but to help shape, mobilize, and combine the vectors which determine the health unit's direction and accountability model so as to bring them closer to the desired system. To shape these forces requires educating the various groups to definitions and demands which are closer to what is legal and ethical and just. This is probably the most difficult part of the creative administrator's job.

Also, for the administrator to mobilize one or more of the relevant groups is to bring about a change in the balance of vectors to which the administrator must later respond. Thus, if the physicians are putting undue pressure on him to take a course of action he considers undesirable, he may instigate a greater activization of the board or of consumer representatives to serve as countervailing forces, somewhat changing the vectorgram. This course can often not be followed because it leads to a measure of counter-mobilization by the other group, in this case the M.D.'s, realizing next to no net change but creating a higher level of conflict all around.[30]

Somewhat better opportunities for creative leadership are open to the administrator in the area of coalition forming. Coalitions arise, not necessarily explicitly, when two or more groups favor the same or a similar course of action. They may be composed of insiders only, outsiders only, or varying combinations. For example, Dr. Lowell Bellin, when First Deputy Commissioner of the New York Department of

Public Health, succeeded in forming a coalition between his agency and the consumers to push a number of voluntary hospitals into giving more resources and attention to ambulatory care.[31] The context was the New York State Ghetto Medicine program which institutionalized the coalition between the public health department and consumers by requiring each hospital desirous of obtaining funds under the program's provisions to (a) subject its ambulatory care services to contractual standard setting, monitoring and enforcement by the New York City Department of Health and (b) to become associated with an Ambulatory Services Advisory Committee, comprising a majority of consumer members. Twenty-two voluntary hospitals in New York City participated in the program. As Bellin et al. note in their *American Journal of Public Health* article, hospital-based ambulatory care services have always been low in the hierarchy of priorities of hospital administrations, in comparison to their inpatient services. Thus the primary incentive for these hospitals to allow their ambulatory care services to be scrutinized by the health department and a consumer group, in marked opposition to their autonomous institutional traditions, was desperation for funds. Yet Bellin et al. also point out that the simple mechanism of a contract between the hospitals and the agency would never have sufficed to insure that the monies earmarked for ambulatory care actually were spent in that manner.

How to prevent the regulated industries from regulating the regulators is a notorious problem in public administration and by itself the agency would never have had the resources to keep the hospitals from reallocating the funds according to their own internal priorities. Though originally skeptical about the value of working with relatively uninformed and inexperienced consumers of hospital ambulatory services, the Department concluded however, that its alliance with the consumers was vital in giving it the leverage which resulted in widespread obedience of contractual stipulations by the hospitals. In addition, quite a number of spinoff improvements in ambulatory care which were not part of the original stipulations were obtained via pressure put on the hospitals by the advisory committees, the Department or the two in concert. In speaking about the accomplishments of the Ghetto Medicine Program, Bellin listed the number of advances that have emerged from this program of active collaboration between consumers and professionals in private voluntary hospitals as follows:

(1) Instituting a unit record system.
(2) Hiring an interpreter.
(3) Establishing a primary physician system.

(4) Developing a list of services for distribution.
(5) Hiring a full-time director of ambulatory care.
(6) Holding two open public hearings.
(7) Adding preventive medicine services.
(8) Assigning additional physicians, nurses, and clerks to the outpatient department.
(9) Eliminating underutilized clinics.
(10) Starting a community outreach program.
(11) Starting a new clinic or other services.
(12) Remodeling clinic and/or emergency room areas.
(13) Running patient attitude surveys.
(14) Providing music and snack machines.
(15) Establishing a communication link between the medical board, administrators, and the consumers.
(16) Changing the referral system.
(17) Changing X-ray and laboratory follow-up.
(18) Extending clinical hours.[32]

The reason coalition building is often effective is that while in isolation each vector is relatively given and unchangeable. On the other hand, the ways in which they may be combined to neutralize, to partially reinforce, or to fully back up one another, is less fixed. The ultimate success lies in building a coalition in favor of greater accountability which is either very wide—or all-inclusive. Then the desired changes are introduced almost as if by themselves.

Closely related, but even more productive, is the formulation of new alternatives. Groups rarely have fully developed positions and almost always can find alternative ways toward their goals.[33] If ways can be found to allow them to advance their goals which at the same time lessen their opposition to other groups and to higher levels of accountability, then the program's success will be particularly pronounced. For example, the strength of the HMO pattern is said to be that it is both responsive to the doctors' legitimate needs and more responsive to the patients than solo practice; if this is the case, it is such a creative alternative.[34]

To advance any or all of these strategies, the administrator needs a considerable understanding of how social systems work, how polities function, what the various groups' values and needs are, and what alternatives are practical and acceptable. In part, he can get the needed knowledge from proper training; in part, from continual interaction with the various groups inside and outside his unit, which impinge on it. Experience suggests that without fixed institutionalized opportunities for communication, such regularized interaction is unlikely to occur with sufficient frequency. The explanation of the mechanisms of institutional communication cannot be undertaken here, but they constitute a vital element of any effective accountability system.[35]

From Unit to System, and the New Definition of Health

So far, we have deliberately followed the prevailing tradition, dealing with the health unit (hospital, clinic, nursing home) as if it were a world unto itself. While the administrator has repeatedly been referred to as dealing with both internal and external forces, those were viewed as impinging on a unit of considerable integrity and cohesiveness. While this view is both necessary (we cannot take in the whole world; we must 'break it up" into units to think about and to deal with it) and favored (especially in non-governmental health units), health units *are* increasingly becoming part of large systems. We do not mean neat, well-consolidated systems, but simply more encompassing entities.[36] Nor is this development necessarily desirable; it may well entail more centralization and more bureaucratization. But, we believe, it is taking place and hence the concern with accountability is, to an increasing extent, a concern with these larger entities.

In part, this is the case because accountability is significantly affected by supervisory, regulatory, "higher order" structures, especially government agencies and professional bodies. In part, this is the case because administrators must manage health systems, not just health units, and the manner in which these are managed greatly affects the performance of the individual units. Last, but equally important, greater accountability in one service area—such as here in health—often requires corrections of ills in other sectors of the society—sanitation, pollution control, highway safety, education—which can only be activated via higher level units or inter unit give and take.

The external factors which affect health have been divided into three categories: (1) technological factors resulting from industrialization, such as air pollution and unsafe working conditions, (2) personal health maintenance factors such as lifestyles encouraging overeating and underexercising, and (3) socio-economic status, especially such health related conditions associated with poverty as inadequate sanitation, overcrowded housing and bad nutrition.

Educational Implications

1. Educational programs which train health administrators but fail to provide them with a set of values to guide their behavior, serve to encourage a lack of accountability. Every program should make as one of its cardinal commitments the development of the normative backbone of the health administrators it trains.[37] To increase the sensitivity of doctors and other health professionals to these matters, Senators Javits, Williams and Mondale have recently submitted bill S 954 which amends the Public Health Service Act to provide "in the training of health professionals, for an increasing emphasis on the ethical, social, legal and moral implications of advances in biomedical research and technology."

This can be achieved only in part via the lecture course. Ethical education may perhaps be best advanced by presenting suitable cases for guided group discussion and through interaction with persons themselves committed to high normative standards. Hence, the faculty entrusted with the education of health administrators needs to include persons of status in this realm, such as clergy who have dealt with dying patients, a hospital ombudsman, a community leader of high standards.

2. The educational program should sensitize future health administrators to the different conceptions of accountability as outlined above. The trainees should come to understand in a deep sense the benefits and drawbacks of passive (or neutral) vs. active (or creative) administration; the limits of morality not backed by social forces; the role of formal factors; the significance, dangers, and limitations of mobilization vs. coalition building, etc. In effect, **in our judgment, the whole preceding analysis is to be viewed as a course outline in accountability,** to be backed up by more extended preparation in appropriate portions of social and political science curricula.

I say appropriate because these disciplines contain segments which are as limited in their perspectives as some of the mono-factorial schools of accountability discussed above. For instance, some stress the role of free will and values per se; others are mesmerized by formal functions, and still others by *Realpolitik*. True, the more a student is exposed and sensitized to even these partial analyses of administration as a social and political system—instead of merely to accounting, financial management, and operations analysis—the more he will understand the processes of accountability and his own range of maneuverability. He may then, maybe with the help of the above outline, piece together his own synthesis. Better still, of course, would be a program built around a social-political science approach which is encompassing and includes the necessary material.

Here again, lectures will do at best only part of the work. Case studies, in conjunction with guided group discussions, backed up with dialogue with experienced administrators would be more helpful. Later in the student's career, a regular (say, weekly) workshop for administrators-in-training, during their "internship" period, might be most effective, because here the participant's own experience can be studied and incorporated as educational experience.

None of these ideas is novel, either as general educational procedure or as efforts in the training of health administrators. Novel would be new systematic combinations, along the suggested lines, for the suggested purposes.

3. The preceding discussion has taken as its cornerstone an implicit assumption which should be explicated, both for the purposes of this presentation and for the purposes of the educational effort we hope will be built around accountability: that the administrator is at the center of the guidance health units and systems and has a leading responsibility for their direction. While special interests are real, the administrator need not be merely the handmaiden of interest groups or a pawn of social forces. Neither is he only on the second string of accountability while doctors man the first line; this is neither reliable nor just. The administrator should have the ultimate responsibility. At the same time, he would be woefully mistaken to see himself as all powerful; an accountable system can arise only through broad support, where the administrator may mobilize, educate, but cannot dictate.

NOTES

1. The Community Health Institute, Health Action Forum #1. November, 1973.
2. Murray Edelman. *The Symbolic Uses of Politics*. Urbana: University of Illinois Press, 1964. Chapter 2.
3. Ibid.
4. Wilbur Rich. "Accountability Indices: The Search for the Philosopher's Touchstone in Mental Health." *Administration in Mental Health*, Fall, 1973, pp. 7–8.
5. For a concrete example of accountability as a rallying slogan in an attempt to build a social movement see Ralph Nader, ed. *The Consumer and Accountability*, for the Center for the Study of Responsive Law. Washington, D.C.: Harcourt Brace, 1973.
6. Avedis Donabedian. *A Guide to Medical Care Administration. Volume II: Medical Care Appraisal*. American Public Health Association, 1969. pp. 100–101.

7. Ibid.
8. Hans J. Morgenthau. *Politics Among Nations.* New York: Knopf, 1954. *Scientific Man vs. Power Politics.* Chicago: University of Chicago Press, Phoenix Edition, 1965. His works are examples of this approach.
9. See Ray Elling. "The Hospital Support Game in Urban Center." Eliot Freidson (ed). *The Hospital in Modern Society.* Glencoe, Ill.: Free Press, 1963. pp. 73–111.
10. See Duncan Neuhauser and Fernand Turiotte. "Costs and Quality of Care in Different Types of Hospitals." *The Annals of the American Academy of Political and Social Science, The Nation's Health: Some Issues,* January 1972. pp. 50–61.
11. Private communication.
12. Charles Perrow. "Goals and Power Structures." Eliot Freidson (ed.). *The Hospital in Modern Society.* Glencoe, Ill.: Free Press, 1963. pp. 112–145.
13. Ibid.
14. David S. Rubsamen. "Doctor and the Law: How Responsible is a Hospital for One of Its Surgeons?" *Medical World News,* February 15, 1974. p. 47.
15. Ibid.
16. Ibid.
17. For more information on this see the chapter entitled Consumer Influence on the Federal Role in *Heal Yourself,* Report of the Citizen Board of Inquiry Into Health Services for Americans.
18. Consumer Notes by Gerald Gold. "The Public Gets Voice in Accreditation of Hospitals. *The New York Times,* December 20, 1973.
19. "HEW Drops Tough Peer Review Plan." *Medical World News,* Oct. 5, 1973. p. 50.
20. For more on this see "The Health Rights Defenders: All Power to the Patients." *Health-Pac Bulletin,* Oct. 1969.
21. Ibid. pp. 2–5.
22. "The Health Rights Defenders: All Power to the Patients." *Health-Pac Bulletin,* Oct. 1969. pp. 2–5.
23. Leonard Broom and Philip Selznick. *Sociology.* New York: Harper and Row, 1963. Third Edition.
24. Ibid. pp. 227–229.
25. For examples and evaluations of more and less successful consumer participation schemes see Jeoffrey B. Gordon. "The Politics of Community Medicine Projects: A Conflict Analysis." *Medical Care,* November–December 1969. Vol. VII, No. 6. pp. 419–428. Roger G. Larson. "Reactions to Social Pressure." *Annual Administrative Reviews of Hospitals,* April 1, 1972. Vol. 46. pp. 181–186. Donna Manderson and Markay Kerr. "Citizen Influence in Health Services Programs." *American Journal of Public Health.* Vol. 61, No. 8. pp. 1518–1523. Frank M. Shepard, M.D. and Beulah Wiley. "A Community-University Cooperative Venture." *Hospitals, J.A.H.A.,* September 16, 1972. Vol. 46. pp. 64–70. Wilfred E. Holton, Peter K. New and Richard M. Messler "Citizen Participation and Conflict" *Administration in Mental Health,* Fall, 1973. pp. 96–103.
26. J. Ehrlich, M. A. Morehead, and R. E. Trussell. *The Quantity, Quality and Costs of Medical and Hospital Care Secured by a Sample of Teamster*

Families in the New York Area. New York: Columbia University School of Public Health and Administrative Medicine, 1962. Quoted in *A Guide to Medical Care Administration, Volume II: Medical Care Appraisal.* American Public Health Association, 1969. p. 110.

27. William R. Meyers, Jane Grisell, et al. "Methods of Measuring Citizen Board Accomplishment in Mental Health and Retardation." *Community Mental Health Journal,* 1972. Vol. 8 (4).
28. For an example of a prototype Comprehensive Health Audit, see Carol Brierly. "Hospital Costs: What the Figures Really Say." *Prism,* February, 1974. pp. 12–17, 62–64.
29. Amitai Etzioni. *The Active Society.* New York: Free Press, 1968.
30. Ibid. Chapters 15, 18.
31. Lowell Eleizer Bellin, Florence Kavaler, and Al Schwartz. "Phase One of Consumer Participation in Policies of 22 Voluntary Hospitals in New York City." *American Journal of Public Health,* October 1972. Volume 62. pp. 1370–1373.
32. Lowell Eleizer Bellin. "How to Make Ambulatory Care Start Ambulating." Presented at the Joint Workshop, sponsored by the AHA and ADAS, Cherry Hill, PA, November, 1971. p. 11.
33. For more on this, see Gabriel A. Almond and G. Bingham Powell, Jr. *Comparative Politics: A Developmental Approach.* Boston: Little, Brown and Co., 1966.
34. For an examination of some of the pros and cons of existing pre-paid programs such as Kaiser-Permanent and HIP see Merwyn R. Greenlick "The Impact of Prepaid Group Practice on American Medical Care: A Critical Evaluation." *The Annals of the American Academy of Political and Social Science, The Nation's Health: Some Issues,* January, 1972. pp. 100–113.
35. For additional discussion see *The Active Society,* chapter 20.
36. On the different types of systems which emerge, see Edward W. Lehman. "Control, Coordination and Crisis: Interorganizational Relations in the Health Field." Center for Policy Research Monograph, 1973.
37. In *Genetic Fix.* New York: Macmillan, 1973, I discuss the formation of a Health Ethics Commission. (Senator Mondale has introduced a bill for the formation of such a commission on the national level). See pp. 183–204, especially.

Roles and Training For Future Health Systems Engineers*

Introduction

In the past few years, health services providers and consumers have become increasingly concerned with the cost, quality and access problems of the health system. Health care costs continue to rise, quality levels of health services are often ill-defined or unacceptable, and access to health care is often inadequately provided.

These problems are typical of service organizations undergoing rapid expansion and philosophical changes in demand for service. In most industries, issues of such a critical nature are addressed by staff specialists.[1] But in health settings, staff members (system engineers, financial experts, data processors, etc.) have been assigned maintenance functions and spend little time addressing critical health delivery system issues. This suggests that staff specialists are not properly utilized in the health field. Several questions arise. Can staff specialists contribute to the solution of critical problems in the health field? What is the appropriate role for staff specialists in health systems? What knowledge, attitudes and skills are needed by staff specialists? What changes are needed to implement these roles? How can these changes be accomplished?

In January 1973, the W. K. Kellogg Foundation through the Com-

---

* by David H. Gustafson, Glenwood L. Rowse, and Nancy J. Howes. This research was supported by contracts from the Commission on Education for Health Administration (the W. K. Kellogg Foundation), the Defense Advanced Research Projects Office and the Office of Naval Research. The authors wish to acknowledge the valuable assistance of Dr. Rockwell Schulz, Mr. Ramesh Shukla, Dr. Charles Pfeiffer, and Ms. Hilde Neujahr of the University of Wisconsin for their help in this study. We also wish to express appreciation to numerous consultants and support personnel for their contributions.

mission on Education for Health Administration, funded a study to address these questions for staff specialists, in general, and health systems engineers (HSEs) in particular. This is a summary of that study. A more complete report is forthcoming. We suggest that interested readers read the complete report since much more detail on both methodology and results can be found there.

Methodology

The questions described above were addressed from two perspectives. One, a traditional approach, identified the problems with how systems engineers (SE's) and other staff specialists are used today and suggested solutions. But a normative approach was also taken. Here consideration of systems engineering was set aside and the major issues facing the health field were identified. Still ignoring systems engineers, the skills, knowledge, and attitudes needed to develop solutions to these problems were determined. Alternate professions possessing these skills were selected. Sometimes systems engineers appeared to be one of the appropriate professions. In these cases existing capabilities were compared to needed capabilities to identify areas of needed improvement.

Three roles for systems engineers were identified from that effort. Knowledge, attitudes, and skills needed to play these roles were identified. Educational requirements for systems engineers and for the users of systems engineers were proposed. Issues of organization, location and use of systems engineers were also addressed.

This study required the input of expertise far beyond that available in the project staff, so numerous consultants were involved in each phase of the study. These ranged from over 240 national experts to identify health systems problems, to 80 practicing systems engineers and 80 users of systems engineers to help appreciate the existing system and test proposed changes, to a multi-disciplinary team of experts to create solutions and review progress of the study. Site visits of both SE programs and educational institutions were conducted to provide a reality base for the study.

Since there is a significant difference between recommending and actually accomplishing change, consultants on social change identified ways to gain recognition for the need for change, bring about reexamination of the SE by the individuals in the health field and provide demonstration projects to test the changes recommended. These were translated into a program for change.

What are the Important Health Care Issues?

Two hundred forty established researchers, new researchers, planners, administrators, physicians, systems engineers, and nurses identified and ranked a list of major barriers (problems) to improving the health care system. Each health professional ranked the barriers according to the amount of positive impact which removal of the barrier would have on the health system, and according to the difficulty and cost involved in doing so.

PROBLEM SELECTION

Those problems most often ranked at the top were compiled into a cluster of most important health system barriers. Each cluster included approximately 15 of the 60 barriers listed for each improvement area (cost, quality, and access); these barriers are listed in Figure 1. On the left of each chart, the number of groups agreeing with the composite list's placement of that item is given. Inter-rater reliability within groups was good but significant differences existed between groups. These are discussed in the full report soon to be published. In order to get a clearer understanding of the barriers, the barriers were separated into categories which seemed to require different knowledge, attitudes, and skills to solve them. These were labeled Operational Problems, Research and Development Problems, Planning and Policy Problems, and Educational Problems.

1. **Operational Problems require the refinement of existing procedures in order to improve productivity or satisfaction in existing health systems.** Projects of this type occur primarily in delivery settings. They focus on techniques for establishing standards, improving work methods and utilization of personnel, planning facilities, developing simple communication and monitoring procedures, and locating and providing needed information for decision makers. Essentially, these are the kinds of projects which traditionally have been and are currently being undertaken by industrial engineers. However, when we grouped the identified high-impact barriers by problem type, *less than 25 percent* of the barriers had components which could be dealt with as operational problems.

2. **Research and Development Problems: Adequate solutions for many problems do not yet exist, and considerable work is needed to develop and test effective solutions.** Such research and development problems were felt to comprise 20 percent of the barriers. These issues

FIGURE 1
Composite List of Important Barriers to Improving the Quality, Cost and Accessibility of Health Care Services

Number of Groups Agreeing*			Barriers	
Access	Cost	Quality		
5	4	7	a)	Consumers lack understanding of preventive measures.
NA	4	7	b)	Consumers lack understanding of when services are needed.
NA	NA	7	c)	Third party payment policies do not adequately discriminate between poor and good quality care.
NA	5	6	d)	Incentives for quality care provided by competitors, governing boards, third party payers, and consumers are minimal.
NA	NA	6	e)	Lack of quality care standards.
4	NA	6	f)	Consumers and providers view service as a reactive rather than a preventive function.
NA	6	5	g)	Organization and coordination of all health services is inadequate.
6	NA	5	h)	Inability to agree on health goals.
NA	4	5	i)	Consumers lack means of providing incentives to improve quality.
NA	NA	5	j)	Needed services are not accessible when needed.
NA	3	5	k)	Consumers hesitate to take issue with the physician.
4	4	4	l)	Information and measures causally relating treatment interventions to outcomes are largely absent.
6	2	4	m)	Fee for service system encourages an increase in the volume of services provided but not in the quality of services.
6	NA	4	n)	Consumers lack understanding of availability of services.
4	4	NA	o)	Providers lack skills to evaluate proposed innovations.
NA	4	NA	p)	Needed cost benefit information does not exist.
NA	3	NA	q)	The increasing and changing nature of demand for health services.
NA	3	NA	r)	Inflation.
NA	2	NA	s)	Implementation skills for cost reduction projects are lacking.
NA	2	NA	t)	Cost reduction projects have had the wrong forms.
NA	2	NA	u)	Providers lack management skills.
7	NA	NA	v)	Consumer problems in financing their health care.
7	NA	NA	w)	Incentives do not exist for physicians to locate in rural or ghetto areas.
6	NA	NA	x)	Services not reimbursed by third party payors are not sought.
6	NA	NA	y)	Legal and educational barriers to use of paramedical personnel.
5	NA	NA	z)	Design skills needed to improve accessibility are not present.
4	NA	NA	aa)	Economic barriers prohibit wide distribution of high cost/low demand services.

* Seven groups responded to quality and access issues (experienced researchers, new researchers, planners, administrators, systems engineers, physicians, and nurses). Physician responses were too few to consider in the cost barriers so the maximum response rate there was six.

have not received much attention outside the walls of academic institutions.

3. **Planning and Policy Problems involve the need for identifying ways to alter the health system at an organization-wide or inter-organization-wide level.** Such problems are tackled primarily in planning agencies and at the corporate planning level. Usually these projects are quite complex and require the use of modeling, considerable data collection, and the interaction and agreement of many diverse types of people. Seventy percent of the barriers had components which could be dealt with as planning and policy problems. Yet, our data analysis suggests that staff specialists rarely address these issues in the health field.

4. **Educational Problems involve the need to improve the knowledge or skills of consumers as well as health professionals.** Fifty percent of the barriers had components which could be considered educational problems. Yet effort directed at educational problems seems to be almost absent in the health system today. Consumer health education is particularly lacking. Although there are inadequate incentives for health agencies to pursue consumer education, apparently the absence of effective techniques for consumer education is equally responsible. Recent success in using a systems approach in developing educational programs[2] suggest that systems engineering may play a role in solving these problems.

What is the SE Doing Today?

A number of studies suggest that systems engineers have not been an effective force in reducing or containing costs, improving quality or improving access to health care.[3,4,5] We accepted these results and set out to determine why. Through site visits, surveys of SE's and SE users and study of the organizational literature we identified five areas that appeared to have played a role in that failure: the problem addressed by SE's, the organizational structure of SE services and the knowledge, attitudes, and skills possessed by SE's.

Over 75 percent of the problems SE's addressed seemed to be operational in nature. This was an important finding because our problem identification studies suggest these are not the central issues. It is also important because it is in conflict with characteristics of successful staff activities in other industries.[6] There, successful staff specialists seemed to address the key agenda items of the governing elites and provide information that would help influence their decisions; issues that in our study appeared to be primarily policy and educational in nature.

Recommendation:

> **Staff specialists in general and systems engineers in particular must attempt to improve their effectiveness in the health field by "penetrating the agendas of the elites" and finding the issues of critical concern. They should address these issues from their unique perspective to provide information with which the elites can improve their decision-making.**

The organization structure of SE programs also seemed to be a major problem. Our research also suggested that a primary concern of staff specialists in the health field was their position in the organizational hierarchy. This was again in conflict with studies of successful staff organizations which suggested that organizational position had very limited impact on staff effectiveness.[7]

Moreover, we found that most SE's were isolated. They were isolated from other disciplines and often addressed problems alone when these problems really required input from many other professionals like sociologists and psychologists. They were professionally isolated from their peers, and so rapidly became obsolete. They were also isolated from the users of SE services by a lack of understanding of critical issues and an inability to communicate. To overcome this problem, Filey and Delbecq found that successful staff groups usually had a boundary spanner to bridge the gap between the elites and the technical staff.[8] Possessing a value system between those of the two groups, the boundary spanner was able to understand and articulate the views of both sides.

Recommendation:

> **Health organizations should have a person who plays the role of boundary spanner between staff specialists and policy makers to communicate with organizational elites and to assign staff to produce information that relates to key issues of concern among elites.**

The systems engineer's knowledge, attitudes, and skills (KAS) also seemed to be a source of difficulty. Although the engineer was technically skilled to address the problems he currently faced, if he began to address critical agenda items of the elites, more sophisticated tools would be needed. Even so, the major weakness seemed to be related to interpersonal incompetence. While inability to talk and write were certainly part of it, a lack of sensitivity to sociopolitical components of decision-making seemed to be equally important. (The section on curricular weaknesses more concretely describes the notable KAS deficiencies of the SE.)

The SE weaknesses presented in this section should not be viewed as a testimonial against systems engineering. SE's have had successes in undertaking improvement projects in the health system. But, for the ultimate benefit of health service systems and consumers, we need to recognize that the potential of SE's has not yet been met. Effort needs to be directed toward understanding and modifying these weaknessses to assist SE's in approaching their potential.

What is the Appropriate SE Role?

The essence of our argument so far is that there are important health delivery problems to be addressed, that specialized problem solving skills are needed to address them, that systems engineers in the field today are not addressing these issues and that given their level of training they are by and large not qualified to address them. In this section we hope to show that SE's properly prepared have an important role to play in addressing these issues.

Problem solving is essentially a change process. A problem is identified, solutions are developed and implemented. If successful the new solution is institutionalized as part of the routine operation of the organization. The role of a systems engineer is then as an agent of change. Research on change is helpful to this study because it provides clues on where the systems engineer can help. Much of that research attempts to identify characteristics that distinguish successful from unsuccessful change efforts. Two things stand out. First, most efforts at problem solving in the health field seem to be characterized by the absence rather than the presence of the success related attributes. Moreover, many SE tools seem to be particularly qualified to bring those attributes to problem solving efforts in health. These are described in detail in Gustafson, Rowse and Howes' full report but some examples will be offered here.

The first phase of Lewin's change process occurs when people recognize and feel a need for change.[9] Utterback's review of the literature suggests that this phase is characterized by several elements.[10] Successful change efforts have information available on losses and benefits of the existing system, etc. SE skills at performance and cost measurement as well as their knowledge of information systems and cost/benefit analysis would seem to be useful here. Successful change programs are also characterized by agreed upon goals and knowledge of the value systems of decision makers. The SE's skill at goal setting and quantification of judgments would seem to be helpful.

The second phase of the change process occurs when new approaches are identified and one is implemented. During this phase of successful programs, problem solving is divided into workable phases and premature closure on solutions is prevented. Each phase of problem solving draws upon different people, etc. Our research suggests these characteristics do not describe problem solving in health. But the SE's tools again seem to be relevant. His problem solving strategy does prevent premature closure and does break problem solving into workable phases. If coupled with group process skills it can draw upon the right people at the right time.

The final phase of change occurs when the new system is evaluated and, if appropriate, is institutionalized. Successful efforts here seem to be characterized by careful planning of implementation efforts, careful analysis of the costs and benefits of the new system, appropriate involvement of other potential users of the change during its test, etc. Our research suggests that in health efforts evaluation is frequently given only lip service and implementation efforts are haphazard. SE tools such as scheduling techniques and program evaluation skills would seem to be helpful here.

This analysis suggests that SE's do have a role in change. It also suggests that the health field might profit by a use of their talents in that effort. Yet we suggest SE's have not done well in the past. Clearly changes in their role and training are needed.

Our research suggests that SE's need to assume three distinct roles in the health field in order to have significant impact. For convenience, these ideal roles are titled *technical facilitator, measurer,* and *modeler.* The three roles have many similarities as all need to receive instruction in engineering as well as behavioral science, in tangible as well as intangible characteristics of systems, and in specific subject content as well as general, universal processes. The technique used by these SE's relate to quantitative and behavioral science measures, problem solving methods, and social interactive methods. All the SE's use a systems approach that breaks problem solving into distinct phases. Their strategies are intended to integrate quantitative and behavioral science techniques from many disciplines in a manner most appropriate to the individual problem. SE's do not complete problem solving by themselves but rather all are trained to use the people most appropriate for each phase in the problem solving effort.

Technical Facilitators

The roles also differ in specific ways: the technical facilitator should first be an expert in catalyzing (technical process facilitating) the development, implementation and evaluation of decision alternatives and, second, should be capable in measurement skills and be able to use modeling skills. He needs to be expert in the catalytic role because decision alternatives are real only if they have been internalized by a critical set of people. For example, literature on social change suggests that internalizing occurs when people feel they themselves have developed the solution. The same literature suggests that several kinds of people are needed at different points in time to develop innovative solutions to problems. Hence, the focus of the facilitator role is to help these people and recognize good decision alternatives.

The development of decision alternatives includes predicting the impact of each alternative. Since measurers or modelers who normally provide this information may not be available, we propose that the technical facilitator should be skilled enough to complete all three basic activities in the role model. Even when measurers or modelers do exist, the facilitator's catalytic tasks will lead him to be a boundary spanner between decision makers and experts, and thus he will have the broadest training of all the SE roles. As such, he should be capable of handling measurement problems with a minimum of assistance and also should be able to identify when modeling is needed, to use existing models, and to manage the development of new ones. In a sense he will become the general practitioner among SE's.

The few SE's who have developed technical facilitator skills have been successful in dealing with problems in many of the health settings described earlier. Among their achievements, at the policy and planning level, have been the design of:

- utilization review programs;
- statewide R&D systems;
- emergency medical service programs;
- a system for improving ambulatory care.

Principal tools of the facilitator include systems design, implementation and evaluation strategies, group process skills, communication skills, scheduling techniques, creative problem solving skills, change process skills, an appreciation of socio-political processes involved in decision making, and a broad understanding of and capability in the full range of systems engineering tools.

Both administrators and SE's occupy roles as agents of change, but their functions and their techniques are quite different. Administrators should be the primary decision makers and should make the socio-political and resource acquisition contributions to the change process. Technical facilitators on the other hand can more appropriately contribute technical process guidance and information. But like all staff specialists and unlike administrators SE's devote full time to using their technical skills in improving the ability of administrators to make good decisions.

The level of skill necessary to undertake the technical facilitator role at the institutional and multi-institutional policy level probably requires graduate training. Undergraduate training may be satisfactory for a person to deal with operational problems in a delivery setting. However, the technical facilitator with long-term managerial interests should also have a master's degree in administration.

Measurers

The measurer should be an expert in the use of measurement to help design, implement and evaluate a program when this expertise is needed at a level beyond that held by the facilitator. He should be an expert in quantifying costs and benefits and in processing this information to assess the impact of decisions (management information systems). He should be capable as a facilitator because a good deal of interpersonal contact (related to process facilitation) is required, and he needs to be strong in group process and communication skills. In addition to his understanding and appreciation of facilitation strategies, he should be able to identfy the need for and to use existing models, especially statistical models.

The measurer would assist implementation efforts by monitoring the process and reporting on its progress to management and providing advice for avoiding potential problems. He can oversee some weaknesses of present engineers by forcing agreement on standards for performing implementation tasks. The measurer also provides (with his expertise in user-oriented information systems) the formal mechanism for monitoring implementation .The measurer can help overcome several common weaknesses of evaluation programs. First, the measurer develops cost and quality measures which make field tests of the new systems more meaningful. Second, he uses statistical quality control methods to predict when the system is likely to experience problems. Third, he uses experimental design techniques to increase the generalizability of findings from field tests so others can benefit from the experience.

The measurer has been successful in dealing with problems at the delivery, policy planning, financing, public health, and R&D levels, including such functions as:

- measuring the relative cost and effectiveness of alternative approaches to organizing and coordinating health services;
- developing and utilizing measures for evaluating the quality of services in a delivery setting;
- measuring personnel efficiency and utilization;
- measuring the cost/effectiveness of delivery systems;
- developing standards of performance for incentive systems to motivate employees; and
- experimentally evaluating the effect of Blue Cross prospective reimbursement for cost of total dental care.

Principal tools used by the measurer include statistical analysis, psychometrics, data sampling, cost/benefit analysis, sensitivity analysis, information systems, and the design of measureable objectives.

The skill needed to assume this role in order to attack operational problems can probably be acquired in an undergraduate degree program. More sophisticated techniques, and thus graduate-level training, are needed to address policy and planning issues at either the institutional or multi-institutional level.

Modelers

The modeler should have expertise in abstracting a health system into a limited but useful set of mathematical elements and manipulating these elements to predict the importance of a decision on that system. These tasks are important in making it possible to evalute a decision before it has to be made and before large amounts of resources are employed to carry out that decision.

Also, because modeling requires an ability to quantify, the modeler must be capable of dealing with complex measurement problems with a minimum of help. He must be a user of facilitation techniques, have (as with other SE's) a thorough understanding of the health field and be competent in interpersonal communication.

The modeler would also develop models to predict the success of implementation strategies. He corrects weaknesses of current change efforts by identifying the environmental constraints that must be kept on schedule if implementation is to be completed on time. Similarly, the modeler contributes to evaluation by creating mathematical models describing alternative systems. Performance of the existing system can be compared with non-existent but possible systems. Since all systems exist only on paper, they can be tested under a broad range of conditions with a relatively small investment.

Modeling has been used successfully in several institutional and multi-institutional planning and policy areas. Among the achievements of modelers examined by our study are:

- allocating funds to construct nursing home bed needs;
- selecting the most cost-effective approach to tuberculosis management for an Indian population;
- deciding whether to implement alternatives to fee for service according to demands for medical services;
- deciding to provide emergency medical services to communities and how to distribute these services, based on accessibility of emergency care;
- developing a model for predicting total hospital costs for a future year, to serve as a basis for reimbursement of costs; and
- developing a model for optimally allocating health maintenance organizations in a metropolitan area.

Tools needed by the modeler are knowledge of modeling, operations research tools, computer programming, and probability theory. To a lesser extent but still important are the tools of data collection and analysis.

Because of the level of skill required before successfully assuming this role, a graduate degree in modeling is probably essential.

Ideal Utilization of SE's

Although descriptions of these three roles might suggest that an SE can function alone in nearly any health setting, such is not the case. The SE needs to be part of a multi-disciplinary team of problem solvers; including not only providers, administrators and SE's but also socio-political planners, finance experts, organization theorists, and (in some cases) experts in behavioral science fields such as sociology, political science, etc.

The SE needs a multi-disciplinary problem-solving team because:

- Health care providers are more sensitive to what it means to manage patient care.

- Planners and administrators are more sensitive to the socio-political factors which influence decision making.
- Planners and administrators are more skilled at bargaining and negotiation.
- The SE will tend to overvalue analytical techniques.
- Financial experts are more skilled in the areas of finance accounting, and economics.
- Behavioral scientists are more sensitive to human values.

In essence, we are saying that systems engineers have a broad set of issues with which to deal. They cannot be expected to function well in all fields (i.e., socio-political, financial, or medical care) so they cannot replace other professionals in the decision making process. To do so would either greatly increase their training time or significantly weaken their strength in systems engineering. However, the technical facilitator by virtue of his systems approach (and catalytic role) is probably the appropriate person to coordinate such a multi-disciplinary team.

Proposed Roles Differ from Present HSE Practice

Engineers working in health settings today fit the technical facilitator role least well. There is some precedent for the technical facilitator role (from its use in the aerospace industry) but the systems strategies used there have not been appropriate for social systems. However, recent advances in systems strategies and group process techniques now appear to have greater relevance to the health field. Unfortunately, few schools currently provide formal training for this role. A few behavioral scientists are beginning to receive training in problem-solving strategies, but they lack capability in the other systems tools needed to complete the technical facilitation role. As a result, very few SE's in the health field today can be described as technical facilitators.

Engineers working in health settings today probably fit the measurer role best. However, our proposed measurer still differs from existing HSE's in two important ways. He differs by a much heavier stress on quantification of judgments and on predictive management information systems. He also differs by the kind of problems he addresses—policy level problems.

The proposed modeler differs from present SE's by his greater concentration on characterizing systems through mathematical terms and developing heuristic solutions to problems (simulation). As a consequence, the modeler places much less emphasis on algorithmic techniques, such as linear programming, than do current operations researchers.

Beyond these differences there are differences in a broad range of additional factors such as knowledge of the health field and interpersonal skills, the present structure and staffing for improvement projects, and the types of problems addressed which must be altered for the proposed roles to be effective. Figures 2 and 3 summarize the proposed roles, now and in the future.

The Problem of Altering Roles

The role modifications recommended above will be difficult to achieve without an understanding of the forces that will be operating for and against the changes. We brought together a multi-disciplinary panel of experts to list those factors. A summary of the analysis of their opinions is given below. Groups interested in modifying SE roles should consult the full analysis in the full report of Gustafson, et al.

THE MEASURER

Two forces seem to favor the proposed measurer role. There does seem to be significant recognition of the need for measurement of cost, quality and access to health services. Moreover, the measurer's role is closest to the way SE's are currently used so it will require fewer alterations in perspectives and attitudes.

But even with increased pressures to measure performance, a number of leaders in the health field will continue to resist pressures to use the measurer role. One reason for this is the lack of proven measures of performance in many areas. Another barrier to speeding acceptance of the measurer role is that one aspect of measurement, management information systems, has been greatly oversold. And, finally, the SE's inability to communicate effectively continues to operate against his success.

THE TECHNICAL FACILITATOR

This role seems to have a great potential for the future. Increasing costs, limited resources, and greater federal control will continue to exert pressure for a more systematic change process. Yet no one seems to be filling this need now. The SE, as an independent staff specialist,

FIGURE 2
Ideal Roles of Systems Engineers — Similarities and Differences

Similarities

* Quantitative and behavioral science training
* Technical facilitation, measurement, and modeling knowledge and skills
* Problem-solving focus
* Systems orientation

General Differences in Emphasis

	Technical Facilitators	Modelers	Measurers
Influence on Decisions	Develop and internalize alternatives	Predict the impact of decisions	Quantify impact of decision (after the fact)
Organizational Position	Process guidance: internal to the changing organization	Model design: external to the changing organization	Data providers: internal or external positions
Interaction with Health Professionals	Direct and frequent interaction at all levels of the changing organization	Indirect interaction through other SEs	Direct and frequent at departmental levels, less so with the "elites" of the organization
Primary Function	*Coordination of technical activities and processes *Guidance, and boundary spanning (general practitioner) *Separation of problem solving into distinct steps *Scheduling the effort *Involving people in the right way	*Prediction through explanation and interpretation of information according to value sets *Developing cost and benefit measures for present and proposed systems *Quantifying the opinions and values of decision makers	*Status levels through collection and aggregation of information *Prediction of process and outcome changes for each decision alternative

FIGURE 3
The Systems Engineer — Present and Future Characteristics

	The SE Today	The SE's of Tomorrow
ROLES	Measurement	Technical Process Facilitation: synthesis of systems and behavioral approaches Measurement: increased emphasis on quantification of judgments and on predictive management information systems Modeling: increased emphasis on mathematical characterization of systems and heuristic approaches
PROBLEMS	Operational	Policy and Planning Consumer Education Operational
SETTINGS	Hospital	Multi-institutional Regional Planning Agencies Regional SE Services Hospitals/HMOs
ORGANIZATIONAL STRUCTURE	Efforts by 1–2 Engineers	Multidisciplinary Teams
INDICATOR OF EFFECTIVENESS	Emphasis on Organizational Position	Emphasis on Agenda of "Elites"
ATTITUDES	Quantification and Systemization Focus on Mastery of Techniques	Quantification and Systemization Problem Focus Flexibility Awareness of Political Influences Concern for the Values of Others
SKILLS	Technical Collection and Analysis of Data	Technical Collection and Analysis of Data Communication or Interaction Skills Implementation Skills
KNOWLEDGE	Traditional Industrial Engineering Tools Structural Knowledge of Health System	More Sophisticated Quantitative Tools for Modeling Systems and Making Decisions Structural Knowledge of Health System Knowledge of Basics Necessary to Manage Patient Care Knowledge of Change Processes and Strategies Knowledge of Sources of Information or Aid Understanding of Social and Political Decision Influences

provides the legitimacy needed to carry out this role. Moreover, the SE does have a history of success as a technical facilitator in other industries and many people suggest that the lack of this skill among health systems engineers is a primary contributor to their past failures.

But this doesn't mean that success will come quickly. There are very few schools that even purport to train technical facilitators and fewer yet that do a good job of it. Real changes in the education of SE's are needed. In addition, since few managers or providers in the health system understand this role concept or are even fully aware of its potential and advantages to them, considerable user education must occur before a technical facilitator would be appropriately used.

THE MODELER

The modeling role will probably be most difficult to implement although there are a number of forces in its favor. First, many leaders in the health field accept the recognition of a need for more rational planning and accept the argument that modeling can help do this. They see that modeling provides them information not now available and they see examples of how modeling has worked in the past. They also recognize that modeling requires special in-depth training. Also supporting this role is the rapidly expanding capability of resources needed for modeling such as computers, data sources, and planning organizations.

But the costs of modeling have been high and past failures have far overshadowed successes. Modeling is a complex process and in certain cases the state of the art in this area has a (long) way to go before it can consistently supply quick and valid predictions from relatively uncostly and obtainable data. Probably most damaging is the negative attitude toward modeling. Many leaders do not understand it, others are threatened by it and others feel that it is impossible to model a process as complex as the processes in the health field.

These factors suggest that real changes are needed before these roles will be successfully implemented. Clearly the systems engineer's education needs to be radically changed. But more than that, health leaders are going to have to want to use SE's and know how to do it properly. For this to happen, the potential of these roles will have to be proven through demonstration projects and effective documentation of results. A corresponding agreement by national opinion leaders to support coordinated implementation will be needed for any rapid widespread change to occur. Then, leaders are going to have to learn how to use staff specialists and both leaders and staff specialists will have to work together to provide the organizational conditions needed for success. Finally, in some areas, such as in modeling and information systems, the costliness of techniques will have to be reduced. The rest of this paper will be spent in detailing these changes.

The Setting

One area in which change must take place is in the settings in which SE's are used. At present, SE's have been employed primarily to attack operational problems in hospitals. However, it is recommended that SE's concentrate their efforts on strategic planning and policy problems which occur primarily in third-party organizations (such as Blue Cross), and planning agencies, and, to a lesser extent, in hospitals. Even in hospitals the critical problems seem to occur at the strategic organization-wide level.

Recommendation:

> Systems engineers should be employed as members of planning staffs, in third party organizations and regional and state health planning agencies. Since this would be a relatively new role for SE's, demonstration programs to evaluate their impact in planning should be conducted. A concerted effort to document and report the results of such tests should be made.

Recommendation:

> Within hospitals, the SE should function primarily, but not solely, at the strategic planning and policy level. Demonstration and documentation of his impact at this level are needed.

Provision of Services: The most common way of obtaining SE services is for a hospital to hire its own full-time SE. This approach has several disadvantages, for the SE quickly gets out of date when there are no other SE's to work with and (even at his best), he cannot be facilitator, measurer, and modeler all at the same time. Moreover, as discussed in the ideal role descriptions, the most creative and effective solutions to major problems are multi-disciplinary in nature. Most SE groups, whether within one hospital or several, have been similarly lacking because they do not possess the full range of SE roles or the other disciplines essential for solving many problems.

Recommendation:

> Systems engineering and other multi-disciplinary health services should be regionalized. A facilitator in each participating organi-

zation (i.e., hospital) would structure problems, identify the need for and manage specialists (such as measurers, modelers, financial experts), and act as a boundary spanner between the specialists team and the organization's own problem-solving group. The team of specialists should operate from a central office and serve a specified group of institutions. Periodically, facilitators should rejoin the central office to maintain a "real world" perspective there as well as to learn new techniques from the team of specialists.

Recommendation:

Several methods of providing regional service are possible. In an urban area, several health delivery organizations or a regional health agency might jointly support a small team of specialists and the facilitator. It might also be possible to subregionalize, with the most commonly used specialists (i.e., measurers, organization theorists, and financial experts) supported locally and the highly specialized experts available on a state or regional level. In this case, modelers might be available through a state agency or through a university extension. Consulting groups might wish to establish such a regional network for the services they offer. All these approachs should be encouraged, evaluated, and reported.

Present Educational Programs for Systems Engineering

Before needed changes in educational programs can be specified and implemented, the characteristics of both ideal and current SE programs must be known. To learn about current programs information was obtained from 26 university engineering programs concerning educational opportunities in health systems engineering.

Telephone interviews were used to obtain information from 20 programs (with a student body of 254), and an additional six more fully developed programs completed a more detailed written questionnaire. Information was sought on: 1) degree alternatives offered, 2) student characteristics and career placement, 3) curriculum emphasis, 4) faculty characteristics, 5) entrance requirements, 6) mechanisms of program evaluation, 7) uniqueness of program, 8) planned program changes, and 9) opportunities for field experience. The detailed results are reported in the Gustafson, et. al., full report. Suffice it to say that these programs have, as with other professions, evolved haphazardly. Few formal degree programs are offered. Most programs emphasized only one role (primarily modeling) in their training. Training in technical facilitation was almost nonexistent. Many faculty professed an interest in the health field, but few were committed to it as their primary research or teaching emphasis. Students were admitted on criteria that predicted academic success but not career success. Very little evaluation of the educational programs was conducted, and the future of these programs was equally uncertain. Some programs planned expansion—others elimination. Almost all programs indicated the importance of field experience but few had a formal program to provide it.

Proposed Educational Changes for HSE's

With the development of more concrete HSE roles, it is felt that the stage is set for significant improvement in the engineer's educational programs. However, if educational changes are to have a significant impact on engineering effectiveness in the near future, our findings indicate that these changes must not only be directed toward HSE's but also toward HSE users and colleagues (other staff specialists on multidisciplinary teams). Equally important to attaining the desired impact is the need to improve inservice or practitioner education as well as the more traditional new career (university) education. The almost negligible attention received in the past by user and practitioner education must be changed. These are imperatives for appropriately and quickly altering the basic roles, skills, and approaches of the many SE's now in the health service system, for continually maintaining widespread competence with rapidly advancing technology, and for providing specialty assistance when required by generalists. Viewed in this way, education should become a lifelong process accompanied by many new methods of provision.

In terms of more specific findings and needed changes, basic characteristics of ideal programs, curricula for the three HSE roles, curricular weaknesses of current HSE and use programs, and recommendations related to instructional settings, curricular packaging, field experience, and selection of students were developed. Although most of the changes are presented in terms of HSE education it is felt that they are generalizable to the education of many other professions.

CHARACTERISTICS OF IDEAL PROGRAM

Literature review and consultant response indicated that educational programs can be characterized in terms of the trends in their outcomes and their processes.

Outcome changes can be predicted in the direction of greater role based education, integration of complementary disciplines, and emphasis placed on skill and attitudinal rather than the traditional knowledge level of learning. The three SE roles proposed in this report provide a basis for beginning to develop more differentiated role based education and beginning to integrate complementary disciplines in educational programs. More specifically, recent research has described several benefits to problem solving efforts which arise from the integration of complementary disciplines emphasizing either behavioral science or analytical engineering approaches.[11] All SE's should receive integrated instruction from complementary disciplines.

The need for increased attitudinal and skill competencies was repeatedly voiced by study respondents. An SE's attitude was felt to be the most important determinant of an individual's success and one of the most common contributions of his failure. In addition, SE weakness in not being able to practically apply or implement his technical knowledge was frequently mentioned. When this is coupled with the continuing knowledge explosion and improving educational methods for dealing with skills and attitudes, it can be predicted that their relative emphasis in curricula will be increased. Even if the emphasis on technical knowledge stabilizes or even decreases, there still will need to be a corresponding increase in practitioner education, high access specialty consultation services for practitioners, or team practice approaches.

Process changes can be predicted for the timing, pacing, and settings of education, the methodologies of instruction, and both student and faculty roles.

In terms of timing and pacing, lifelong career education will be stressed. An increasing range of refresher courses, practicums, seminars, and "new topic" courses will be offered to practitioners when they have a specific need. In this, attempts will consciously be made to integrate the practitioners' needs with the theoreticians' developments. And, the emphasis now placed on initial degrees will be diminished with competency levels, determined by a combination of experience and formal training maintained throughout one's career, being stressed.

Career education presents an educational access problem to geographically constrained practitioners. This problem will require educational services to decentralize or at least to develop better links between the two groups. Regionalized services, improved extension services, and "inhouse" training programs are all likely to be developed.

There are many valid instructional methods available, yet rarely is more than one used for any given unit of instruction. To effectively individualize instruction to meet the content and locational needs of each practitioner or student, flexibility must become a descriptor of instruction. The semester approach will gradually lose its dominance with curricular decision points becoming more frequent and occurring at different times for different students. Units of instruction will in turn become smaller and more packaged to permit the desired flexibility, as well as more controlled and effective instructional design and measurement. Greater use of resources in the community will be used to facilitate individualization. Individualization will also necessitate a move from group referenced to criterion referenced evaluation of students. Although more difficult, they permit both individual evaluation and precise quality measures of learning, whereas the traditional group-referenced assessments do not.

As the specification of specific methods for individual students has not been consistently successful in the past (Jamison et al., 1974), another strategy should predominate for a time. The strategy which has been more successful (in terms of both improved learning levels and satisfaction) is the provision of multiple alternatives by which each of the conditions for successful learning could be met and then leaving most (not all) of the selection decisions to the student.[12] This strategy should be complemented by rigorous content selection[13] and appropriate goal setting procedures for students[14] since these factors have been found to have as much or more of an impact on learning outcomes as does the selection of specific instructional methods.

Student and faculty roles are both expected to change significantly in the future. Students will make many more decisions on their own. They must take the initiative to use information resources which improve their decisions. Faculty members must take the initiative to improve both information resources related to instructional alternatives, possible career paths and career opportunities and mechanisms which evaluate an individual student's strengths and weaknesses in relation to his goals.

The ideal changes which have been described are expected in the distant future—15 to 20 years (Commission on Nontraditional Education, 1973). From our review of current systems engineering programs, it is apparent that few, if any, of these changes are being seriously developed at this time. The changes described are important. If university structures cannot adapt to these needs, then other educational providers must be given the opportunity to do so.

Curricula for HSE's

After identifying critical health system problems, a multi-disciplinary team including SE's, educators, health professionals, and representatives from relevant disciplines identified solutions sets and their related knowledge, attitudes, and skill (KAS) sets needed to attack the major problems. A comprehensive KAS set was developed and presented to health service administrators and practicing SE's around the country who rated the items according to their importance to SE success for each of the three proposed roles. These ratings were refined by staff and consultants for use as educational objectives. Knowledge, attitude, and skill objectives were developed for role related information, information collection techniques, specialized information processing (human factors engineering, facilities design, job analysis), statistical tools, operations research, decision analysis, management information systems, formal change processes (design, implementation, and evaluation), formal communication processes, social system sciences, health system characteristics, and computer technology. A crosscheck was made to insure that objectives existed for functional topics, application topics, and integrative or relevancy topics wherever appropriate. The complete list, ratings by item of the competency level needed by each role, and core ratings for all three SE roles, may be found in the full report of Gustafson, et al.

When the ratings were examined by our staff and consultants and integrated with site visit data, the following global recommendations relating HSE roles to depth of training were developed:

Recommendation:

> Persons interested in addressing *operational problems* do not need graduate preparation in systems engineering. But, they do need a thorough understanding of the health field. These people should have a baccalaureate degree in Industrial/Systems Engineering, and a Masters in Health Administration. They should assume positions on the administrative staff of delivery institutions. Programs in Health Administration should increase recruitment of students with this undergraduate background.

Recommendation:

> Individuals interested in strategic planning and policy issues need more knowledge, attitudes, and skills than can be obtained from undergraduate programs. Thus, masters degree programs in industrial/system engineering with training in the health system should be developed for the three SE roles. Since the technical

facilitator's role (because of its boundary spanning nature) needs greater in-depth understanding of health as well as sociopolitical processes, individuals interested in this role should pursue a combined masters program in IE/systems and either health administration or health planning.

Recommendation:

Persons interested in addressing problems of consumer education in health need a background in educational strategies as well as systems engineering. Programs should be developed that offer a dual masters program in systems engineering and education. Thus, a part of the systems training should also include background sources in the health field.

Recommendation:

Individuals interested in R&D issues in health systems engineering need a Ph.D. level education. Centers of excellence, in not only systems engineering and health, but also in a broad range of related disciplines (economics, psychology, statistics, computer science, organization theory, sociology) should be encouraged to develop such programs as part of an overall effort in health services research.

CURRICULAR WEAKNESSES

When the developed educational objectives were compared with responses to our educational program questionnaire, characteristics of our site visit of HSE's and ratings from 80 health administrators and 80 practicing SE's, several areas of needed instruction were identified as being seriously underattended.

1. **Attitudes.** Our data indicated that the experts felt attitudinal characteristics were of greater importance to the engineer's success than either his skills or his knowledge. In addition, three of the five greatest SE weaknesses rated were attitudes. Despite these ratings, the educational programs surveyed gave only hit-and-miss attention to a few attitudes. The most important and common attitudinal weaknesses of practicing engineers were found to be:

- Inflexibility of engineers.
- Lack of real acceptance that the political process is an important part of social change.
- Inadequate concern by engineers for the agendas of decision making "elites."

- Lack of recognition that many analytical and organizational techniques have significant limitation in the real world.
- Minimal feeling placed by engineers on the values, ideas, and feelings of others.

Hoos in her analysis of SE's in public policy also suggested these weaknesses.[15]

2. **Knowledge and Skills.** SE's seem to be fairly strong in traditional tools. These tools work well with operational problems but for policy level problems a greater level of sophistication is required. This sophistication relates to the more complex quantitative tools for measuring benefits, forecasting trends, and modeling systems. Most HSE's currently lack this sophistication. This weakness, however, is relatively minor and easily dealt with when compared to weaknesses in those skills and knowledge that support the use of systems tools. The most important qualifications found to be lacking were, respectively:

- Communication or interaction skills.
- Skills permitting the application of theory to real problems.
- Integrated knowledge—of one tool with another and of theory with practice.
- Factual knowledge about the health services system.
- Understanding of change processes and implementation skills.
- Knowledge of sources of information or aid.
- Understanding of decision influences—particularly political and social influences.
- Knowledge of ideal HSE roles.

These are the areas needing curricular modifications whether they require simple strengthening of courses or the addition of new techniques or units of instruction such as field experience to deal with application and interpersonal skills or self-contained modules to insure that attention is given to attitudes, integration or relevancy objectives, and interpersonal skills. It should be evident that knowledge of how to use a technique, while important, is not sufficient. It should also be clear that we feel *the educational system has failed to equip the SE with the necessary adjuncts to that technical education.*

3. **User Education.** To effectively support and contribute to the SE's efforts, managers and users of engineering services must value SE goals and understand their roles, techniques, and jargon well enough to appreciate and interact with SE's. Yet, ineffective organization and

use of engineers was common in our site visits and at least partly due to this lack of understanding. To make matters worse practitioners are receiving almost no user education.

Even in universities, health administration programs have only offered some user instruction (in quantitative methods) to their students. Even that focus has been too narrow; the wrong tools have been focused on, and the expectations of students have been inappropriate. First, the focus has been too narrow because a broad range of SE capabilities (including the systems approach, decision analysis, and predictive information systems) have been missing. Second, many of the tools covered (primarily those associated with mathematical programming) can only be justified for very few problems and even then under quite restrictive assumptions. Consequently, these tools should receive less attention in health administration programs. Third, these courses are taught as if the student were expected to develop some level of proficiency in the content of them. Instead of this, the courses should develop in the student a capability to understand and properly use the SE staff specialist as well as an understanding of how to use a set of tools. To do this, students need to understand SE roles, potentials and weaknesses. Where tools must be taught the student should learn only their function, strengths and weaknesses.

Recommendation:

> To increase the impact of systems engineering on the health system, it is recommended that formal methods for providing and encouraging user education be developed.

Educational Settings

Three of our proposed educational changes have significant implications for educational settings. These recommended changes are 1) the development of coordinated lifelong career education for HSE practitioners, 2) the development of SE user education, and 3) the provision of multiple instructional alternatives which effectively integrate learning objectives with learning theory and individual student needs.

Information obtained from site visits and consultants suggests that existing educational settings are not fulfilling these needs because the educational opportunities provided are not sufficiently accessible to SE practitioners and users, the educational opportunities provided do not sufficiently meet learning or learning style needs of present or future SE practitioners and users, and effective linking or coordination does not occur across the settings.

Recommendation:
> Many different educational settings and instruction methods are needed to meet all the individual needs of future and present SE practitioners and users. Specifically, new delivery services and settings need to be developed and evaluated for the regional or local needs of SE practitioners and users. These new services must be accessible for use in or near the professional's home or work place, and must be oriented to the characteristics of individual adult learners (e.g., meeting needs when they occur and according to an individual's learning style). They must also be recognized and valued by employers before incentives and resources for their use will be sufficiently present.

Recommendation:
> In order to effectively meet the learning needs of practitioners, considerable development is necessary to organize small learning units around frequent difficulties encountered by SE practitioners and users and around priority health problems. These units must place greater emphasis on application skills and strategies than on theoretical concepts.

At present, career education (as it progresses through undergraduate, graduate and continuing education) has almost no systematic coordination. Consequently, many services are underdeveloped and students receive almost no guidance in planning their career education or in identifying and using available services. Even within universities, intentional coordination and cooperation across departments is felt to be minimal.

Recommendation:
> Development and demonstration projects need to be undertaken to improve planning and policy, and continuing education services and to coordinate the entire educational system for HSE career education. This must include the formal organizations and acceptance of this delegation by all other educational organizations.

Recommendation:
> Formal recognition of a person's achievements both in formal education and through work experience is needed to upgrade the quality of SE's. Methods should be developed by universities so that degree credit is given for work experiences and related courses in other disciplines or universities. Where possible, residency requirements for degrees should be severely reduced if not eliminated.

Recommendation:

The value of a national record of competency to record the knowledge, attitudes, and skills developed by an individual SE over time should be evaluated. The record should be voluntary but should make an SE's records available to employers. Its intent is to provide incentives for continued development of an SE's competencies. It should not be developed in a way which stifles the use or flexibility of engineers by the differential labeling of individuals.

UNIVERSITY DEPARTMENTAL ORGANIZATION

The educational changes proposed thus far are both many and costly, requiring considerable justification for developmental efforts. Within university programs an average of less than six health oriented students (as reported by existing SE programs) certainly would not provide the needed critical mass for independent development. So the authors feel certain that a degree department of health systems engineering should not be developed. Yet we feel that health systems engineers need an education different from those working in manufacturing since the values, problems, and issues of the two industries differ and the tools, measurements and objectives functions employed are different. On the other hand, however, the values and tools of HSE's may not be significantly different from those of a criminal justice SE or an educational SE, etc. There may be value to developing a human services engineering program that trains people to address systems problems in human service industries such as health systems, criminal justice, education, welfare, waste disposal, etc. The development of a human services engineering department would easily permit the gathering of a critical mass of students in order to justify obtaining all of the resources needed for quality educational programs.

More globally, human services departments should be oriented around basic functional topics as are all functional departments (e.g., engineering, administration, planning, sociology, economics). To prepare individuals for roles, these departments must draw upon application clusters such as health systems, criminal justice, education, etc. These application clusters might be considered departments but should not be degree granting entities. A health system cluster would prepare individuals from all types of functional disciplines who desire careers in the health system. Consequently, the staff of application departments would be comprised of many diverse professors each holding a joint appointment in Health Systems and in one of the functional departments. The purpose of application departments would be multidisciplinary integration, provision of application information and the development of application skills. Consequently, these departments could assume the responsibility for coordinating field experiences and could require a different type of faculty role (integrative) than do functional departments (theorists). Thus, it is recommended that:

> **A study of the need for a new program of human services engineering should be conducted.**
> **A core of service related information courses should be developed for the area of health as well as for criminal justice, education, etc. Students from all functional disciplines (engineering, administration, planning, sociology, economics, social work, etc.) should be able to draw from these courses but no degree should be given in them specifically.**

Curricular Packaging

It will not be easy to provide for a system of quality education that is available in every community and that gives recognition of the achievements made by all students. However, several structural options exist; among them are the AHEC (Area Health Education Center) and open university and national university concepts. In each case, self-contained educational modules need to be developed for these options to be feasible. If these modules are individualized so that students in several environments can use them effectively, quality education can be provided anywhere and anytime in an engineer's career.

Equally important is the impact which these modules can have on the overall quality of education. Today, educational systems (including HSE programs) have many students with diverse characteristics, ever expanding knowledge bases from which to teach, and numerous diverse responsibilities placed upon faculty members. HSE educational programs are also characterized by incomplete curriculum and instructional development. The authors feel that self-contained modules can help to "individualize instruction, standardize learning levels, expand curricular offerings, meet practitioner needs, and control management problems by establishing and packaging":

- small units of knowledge,
- alternative instructional procedures, and
- standard management policies

for students with different learning needs, learning styles, and personal needs. Once packaged only minimal effort is required for faculty members to re-use or improve a unit of instruction.

If modules were developed, students in almost any location could pick up one of these packaged units and expect to effectively attain knowledge or skills by appropriately choosing one of the alternative instructional procedures for which needed resources (e.g., texts, workbooks, group members, preceptors) were available. Modules can also be developed around practitioner needs, so a convenient vehicle exists for the improvement of practitioner education.

Module development is a very feasible strategy for controlling and improving the quality of educational programs, both because modules can be developed incrementally for recognized areas of weakness in the program and because the standardization of modules facilitates further evaluation and improvement of the modules themselves. The integration, attitudinal, and information source modules suggested earlier are examples of weak curricular areas for which modules could be easily developed.

Even though the need for modules may be realized, the development of modules is not a simple task. The contributions of subject specialists, educational process specialists, and potential users must all be attained in order to develop modules which are effective, enjoyable, and creative enough for students and faculty members to want to use them. In addition, it takes considerable time and funds to develop even a few hours of quality modules. Thus, if modules are to be developed in any quantity, it seems that a coordinated national developmental effort is required along with distribution of modules developed by any participating institution.

Because of the benefits which accrue from modules and the problems which arise from the development of modules, the following strategy to develop modules is recommended:

> **A coordinated nationwide effort should be undertaken to develop and distribute a broad range of high quality educational modules on health and systems engineering topics. Where possible, these modules should be flexible enough to permit individuals in several environments to use them, and responsive enough to permit and encourage use not only for planned needs but in response to unplanned needs of practitioners.**

Field Experience

Field experience can, if properly provided, be a critical part of a student's education. It can serve to orient students to the health system, help students internalize important attitudes, and skills, and help students integrate and apply the theoretical training they have received.

Unfortunately since it could deal with some of the important SE weaknesses identified, few SE programs have adequate field experiences for their students. A caution is needed since quality field experience for many students is very difficult to provide. They can be so powerful that a traditional preceptor can easily overshadow the more passive learning of the classroom wherein the student is being trained for tomorrow not for today. Consequently, it seems best to encourage a few centers of excellence for field experience in order to refine the art and to ensure quality. For those developing field experiences, a few guidelines to providing quality experiences are: separate experiences into distinct components for distinct objectives tied to the theoretical knowledge being developed vicariously, periodically offer appropriate experiences after formal theoretical instruction, obtain progressive preceptors, and develop frequent regularly scheduled meetings between the preceptor, student, and faculty member.

Recommendation:

Preceptorships and field experiences need to be integrated with the formal core of the educational program and an educational strategy to achieve this must be developed. Preceptors must make a commitment of both time and energy, and a few centers of excellence for field experience should be encouraged and supported.

SELECTION OF STUDENTS

The selection of students for an educational program must match student characteristics with requirements for success in a specified role after graduation from the program as well as with requirements for completion of the educational program. Success in a role is influenced by factors external to the engineer (characteristics of the situation or setting) and by factors internal to the engineer (his knowledge, attitude and skill characteristics). Characteristics of the engineer include elements which are learned in educational programs or early in the job experience and elements which are more permanent cognitive and personality traits that are not appreciably changed or taught in educational programs. The latter traits are the crucial selection criteria.[16] At this time, they have only partially been identified and separated from situational and trainable influences on engineering success. Elements of situational influences included such things as physical demands of the setting, proximity of resources, attitudes and values of working colleagues, legitimacy required, stage of the project and problem type.

From information we were able to gather we have concluded that:
- Selection methods of current educational programs effectively predict academic success but not on-the-job success.
- Selection criteria must vary for the measurement, modeling and technical facilitation role emphases. In addition, graduate students should be guided to accept positions only in settings or situations compatible with their personal characteristics.

It is recommended that:

Research should be undertaken to develop and demonstrate more effective student selection methods. Both complex testing techniques and the simpler checklist type strategies should be pursued.

Students with prior health experiences should be given preference in admission to graduate level SE programs both to insure higher quality students and to encourage the improvement of current practitioners. Due to financial burdens on those who have been in the field for some time they may need financial support before they can be convinced to apply.

Crucial elements in SE job success appear to be: basic, intellectual ability (not necessarily high), basic technical skills, optimism, creativity tendency, high energy level (self starter), personable with and perceptive of the needs of all types of people, tendency toward self evaluation, and focused personal interests which contribute to role success. Greater specification of these selection criteria is needed.

Improvement of Health Systems Engineering: The Next Step

Among all the changes which have been discussed for improving engineering impact on the health system, three foci for change stand out. The most central is the modification or separation of current health systems engineering roles. Without acceptance of this need, the other changes will not readily follow or have significant impact. The second focus should be improvement in the levels of current and future competencies of SE's. In order to improve SE impact on the health system in the near future, the third focus should be establishment of educational opportunities focused at SE users and SE practitioners rather than at improvement of initial training programs. In turn, implementation of these changes will necessitate significant reorganization of the provision of SE services to the health system and alteration in the objectives and methods of educational programs. This section proposes a specific strategy for beginning to implement all of the recommended changes. It is not a complete strategy but instead elicits support for these changes and provides a mechanism for completing development of the strategy.

Implementation of new HSE roles can progress either through a comprehensive nationally coordinated activity or through sporadic efforts to demonstrate the need or value of new methods which in turn catalize the next level of sporadic development and demonstration projects. Although the first type of activity should produce more widespread and effective implementation in a shorter period of time, it does require some initial development and demonstration before national opinion leaders will have the incentive to support a nationally coordinated implementation activity.

Catalyzing the Change Process

It is proposed that nationwide support for change in HSE roles can be developed by a carefully run conference attended by opinion leaders in systems engineering, health systems, and related disciplines and application areas.

Recommendation:

> **A conference, bringing together no more than 100 opinion leaders in systems engineering and the health field as well as relevant speciality experts, should be held as soon as possible. The purpose of this conference should be to discuss and if possible agree upon the need for separation of health systems engineering into three distinct roles, then, if this need is agreed upon, to discuss the other changes recommended in this report and establish a national committee for coordinating development and implementation of needed changes.**

In addition to a broad consensus supporting and defining the needed change areas, products of this conference should be priorities on needed changes, initial strategies for developing or implementing these changes, the appointment of a national committee for coordinating implementation activities after the conference is ended, attendee commitments to future activity, and a book describing the results of the conference.

Figure 4 presents an overview of the implementation strategy which has been described. Its dominant characteristic is the intended obtain-

FIGURE 4
Verification and Implementation of a New Health Systems Engineering Role

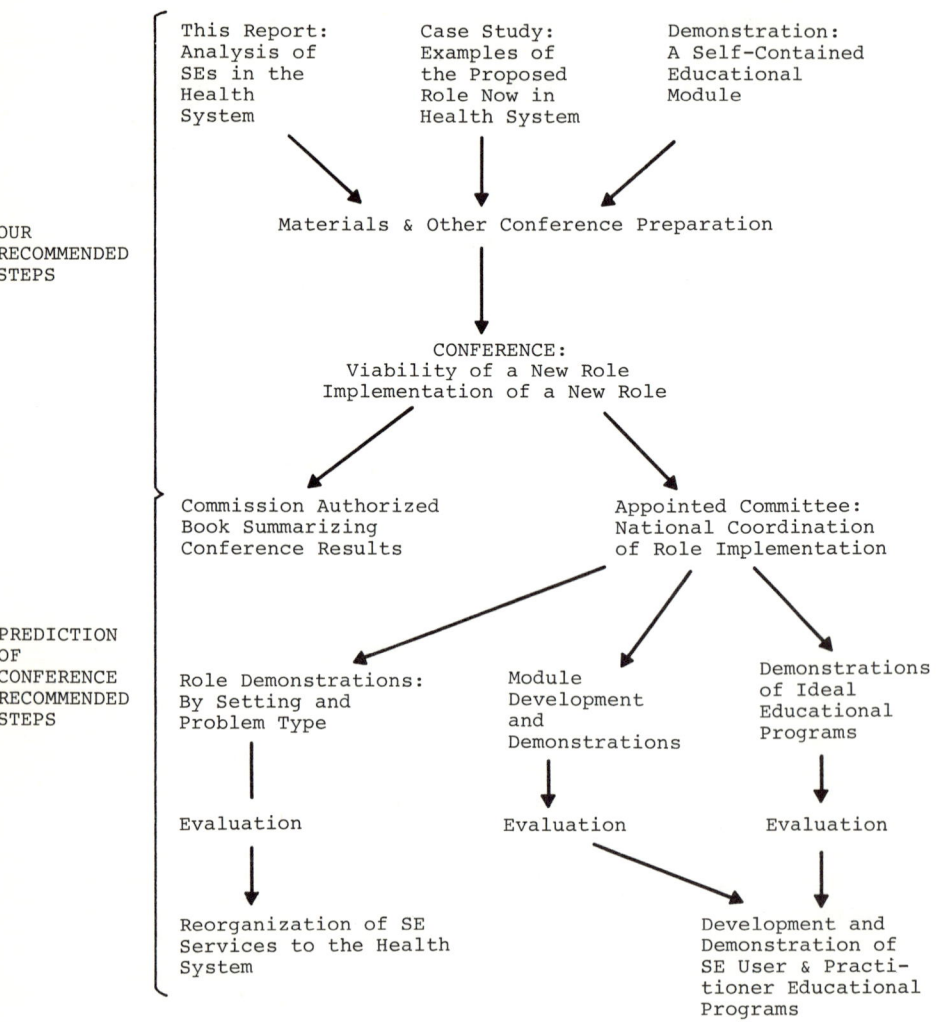

ment of a cooperative national change effort. Any of the individual development and demonstration projects which represents a part of this strategy can be undertaken with the expectation of beneficial outcomes. However, the resultant influences (of a piecemeal strategy) during the next ten plus years is minimal when compared with the influence which the conference strategy should have during the next ten plus years.

Notes

1. Gerold Hage and M. Aiken. "Social Change in Complex Organizations." New York: Random House, 1970.
2. M. Vere DeVault and J. Kean. *Wisconsin Elementary Teacher Education Project.* Washington, D.C.: U.S. Dept. of Health, Education and Welfare, 1969.
3. D. Stimson and R. Stimson. *Operations Research in Hospitals: Diagnosis and Prognosis.* Chicago: Hospital Research and Educational Trust, 1972.
4. J. Freeman and R. Gue. "Information Systems and Operations Research in Health Care." A paper presented to the 2nd ORSA Health Applications Section Symposium; "Health Operations Research; a Critical Analysis." Atlantic City, New Jersey. November 9, 1972.
5. C. Hardwick and H. Wolfe. "Incentive Reimbursement/Industrial Engineering Experiment." Chicago: Blue Cross Association, 1970.
6. Donald C. Pelz and Frank M. Andrews. *Scientists in Organizations.* New York: Wiley and Sons, 1966.
7. Hage, op. cit.
8. A. Filey and A. Delbecq. "Program and Project Management in a Matrix Organization: A Case Study." University of Wisconsin, Madison: Bureau of Business Research and Services, Monograph #9, Chapter 3. 1974.
9. Kurt Lewin. "Group Decision and Social Change." G. E. Swanson, et al. *Readings in Social Psychology.* New York: Henry Holt & Co., 1952. pp. 459–473.
10. James M. Utterback. "Innovation in Industry and the Diffusion of Technology." *Science,* Feb. 15, 1974. Vol. 183. pp. 620–626.
11. K. A. Archibald. "Three Views of the Expert's Role in Policy-making: Systems Analysis, Incrementalism, and the Clinical Approach." *Policy Sciences,* January 1970. pp. 73–86.
12. R. Dubin and T. Taveggia. "The Teaching-Learning Paradox: A Comparative Analysis of College Teaching Methods." Eugene: Center for the Advanced Study of Educational Administration, University of Oregon, 1968.
13. Decker F. Walker and Jon Schaffarzick. "Comparing Curricula." *Review of Educational Research,* Winter, 1974. Vol. 44, #1.

14. E. Locke and J. Bryan. "Grade Goals as Determinants of Academic Achievement." *Journal of Psychology,* 1968. Vol. 29. pp. 217–228. E. Locke, N. Cartlege and C. Kneer. "Studies of the Relationship Between Satisfaction, Goalsetting, and Performance." *Organizational Behavior and Human Performance,* 1970. Vol. 5.
15. Ida Hoos. *Systems Analysis in Policy Planning.* Berkeley: University of California Press, 1972.
16. John P. Campbell, et al. *Managerial Behavior: Performance and Effectiveness.* New York: McGraw-Hill, 1970.

The Demand for Hospital Administrators[*]

Introduction

Stimulated by the growth of hospital and medical insurance, the health services sector has been the most rapidly growing sector of the American economy for 40 years. Employment, investment, output, and prices have consistently grown more rapidly in the health field than in any other. Our next great social reform, national health insurance, will attempt to make the benefits of health service available to our entire population by eliminating geographical and financial barriers to access. Will this reform further stimulate growth, retard it, or leave it unaffected? We attempt, here, to provide part of the answer to this important question.

We project only the demand for primary and secondary administrators of hospitals. These are a small minority of all health administrators, an occupation that includes administrators of nursing homes, health insurance plans, public health programs, health planning agencies, and many other related activities. The limits of our study were wholly practical. In order to estimate the demand functions on which our forecasts rest, we needed detailed information about individual administrators and the institutions that employ them. In the case of hospital administrators we were able to link together records provided by the American College of Hospital Administrators and by the American Hospital Association to get the needed data. The Medical Group Management Association provided us with equivalent data for managers of medical groups. These M.G.M.A. data were used to trace

---

[*] by Roger Feldman and Richard N. Rossett. This paper is a shortened version of a paper prepared for the Commission with support from the Kellogg Foundation. The authors gratefully acknowledge that support as well as the generosity of the American Hospital Association, the American College of Hospital Administrators, and the Medical Group Management Association, all of whom provided data employed in the study on which this version is based.

the effects of a large-scale program of establishing H.M.O's on the demand for hospital administrators. Though the demand for medical group administrators was examined, projections of demand for them depend trivially on population forecasts, so no projections were made. Though other professional associations were willing to provide us with data, in no other case were we able to construct the necessary records linking employee to employer.

We confined our study to the demand for administrators and ignored the supply side of the market because our forecasts of demand growth proved so modest as to be well within the ability of the market to accommodate, even under our most extreme assumptions. An element often overlooked by forecasters is the mechanisms by which discrepancies in rates of growth of supply and demand are adjusted by market forces. Some factors that affect supply and demand may be growing at rates that produce widening shortages or surpluses when they are projected into the future. From Malthus to the Club of Rome, such naive projections have produced alarming predictions of catastrophe. But we should remember that prices (in this case, salaries paid to administrators) will rise to stimulate entry into the profession when there is a shortage and will fall to discourage entry when there is a surplus. Had our forecasts shown either remarkable increases or decreases in the demand for administrators, we then would have needed to estimate the supply function as well as the price adjusment function. Since we forecast only modest increases, these steps were unnecessary.

The Demand for Hospital Administrators

The demand for hospital administrators is a derived demand, depending on the primary demand for hospital services. Since the demand for hospital services will be affected by the establishment of national health insurance, a forecast of the demand for administrators must rest on a forecast of the primary demand. Two distinct demand functions must be employed in calculating each forecast: a function in which characteristics of the hospital determine how many administrators it will hire and the level of training it will require, and a function in which income, insurance coverage, and demographic characteristics determine the price people will pay for hospital care. Experience in the United States has shown that increases in the demand for hospitalization tend to result in increases in quality and sophistication of service accompanied by price increases, rather than by expansion of hospital bed capacity. For this reason we take price, as determined by the demand for hospitalization, as an input variable in the hospital's demand function for administrators. The higher the quality of service a hospital offers and the more sophisticated it is, the more administration it will require and the more skill and training the administrator must have.

Three sorts of hospital demand functions were estimated: one predicts the number of administrators a hospital will employ (usually either one or two, where the definition of an administrator simply depends on whether he is eligible for membership in the A.C.H.A.), the second predicts his level of education (B.A., M.A., M.B.A., Ph.D., M.D., etc.), and the third predicts whether his training will have included special training for medical administration (as in a hospital administration program rather than in a business administration program). Ideally, a single demand function should be estimated that would predict, simultaneously, the number of administrators, their levels of education, and whether or not they received special training, but neither the data nor the present state of statistical methodology permitted us to satisfy all these objectives.

Even so, the statistical methods employed had to be specially selected to suit the somewhat unusual problem confronted here. Two of the demand functions had categories rather than continuous quantities as their dependent variables. This meant that a special technique, probit analysis, had to be employed. This is a technique, derived from biological assay, that permits estimation of an equation from which it is possible to calculate the probability that an individual case will fall into each of several categories, given the values of variables that affect the probability. In the case of several levels of education, hospital variables like total number of admissions, number of beds, expense per patient day, and number of employees are used to predict the probability that the administrator will have, say, a B.A., an M.A., or some higher degree. This equation can be used to predict, for 1,000 hospitals, how many will employ administrators of each type.

Even the equation for the number of administrators is of this type, since a hospital can employ an integral number of administrators, but not fractions of administrators. Probit analysis was used to estimate all three types of demand functions.

In all, six demand functions for hospital administrators were estimated, since for each of the three types of functions, one was estimated for chief executive officers, and one for secondary administrators.

Using A.H.A. and A.C.H.A. data, we had 2,989 cases of hospitals that employed either one (2,807 cases) or two (182 cases) chief executive officers, and 1,158 hospitals that employed, 1, 2, 3, 4, 5, or 6 + secondary administrators (666, 312, 113, 37, 17, and 13 cases respectively). The number of hospitals was less than half the number listed by the A.H.A. guide issue and the number of administrators in our sample is only about one third of all primary and secondary administrators presently employed by hospitals. The fact that not all administrators who are eligible for membership belong to A.C.H.A., combined with problems of incomplete records make it impossible to base our study on the entire universe. Still, as a partial check on our equations, we used all the A.H.A. hospital records together with our estimated equations to estimate the total number of administrators in 1971, the year to which our data pertain. Our estimate is that in 1971 there were approximately 16.5 thousand primary and secondary administrators employed in hospitals in the United States.

Salient features of the demand equations were as follows:

1. The number of administrators employed by a hospital, both primary and secondary, is determined almost entirely by the number of admissions, with teaching hospitals tending somewhat to employ more than non-teaching hospitals.

2. The total number of beds and the expense per patient day are the two factors most important in determining the level of education of a chief executive officer, with increases in either tending to increase the level of education demanded. In the case of secondary administrators, expense per patient day is important, but not admissions.

3. For both sorts of administrators, high admissions is associated with specialized training in medical administration. Only for the chief executive officer is expense-per-patient day strongly related to the probability of specialized training, though the relationship is positive for both types of administrator.

The Demand for Medical Group Administrators

Few medical group administrators have had specialized training in medical administration (two percent in our sample) so analysis based on that classification is of little value. The analysis of factors that determine the number of administrators employed by a medical group and their levels of education was done in the same way as analysis of hospital administrators except that no distinction was made, because of data limitations, between chief executive officers and secondary administrators. Again, the definition of an administrator was simply eligibility for membership in a professional association, in this case the Medical Group Management Association, which kindly supplied us with the data. Three types of demand function were estimated: one predicting the number of administrators (ranging from 1 to 4 per group, with frequencies of 718, 54, 8, and 4 in our sample), another predicting the type of degree, and a third predicting the number of years of schooling. Three factors proved significant in these demand functions: the more hospital beds controlled by a group, the more education they demanded for their administrators; if the group was an H.M.O. it demanded more education than if it was not; and the more full-time physicians participating in the group, the more administrators it employed.

The Demand for Hospitalization

A demand function estimated by Martin Feldstein [1971] was used to predict hospital prices which were used, in turn, to predict hospital demand for administrators. Feldstein found that the price that will equilibrate the supply and demand for hospitalization is a function of per capita disposable income, population density, the ratio of primary care physicians to population, and the level of hospital insurance coverage. The first three of these factors were projected through the use of simple models designed to reflect some of the complexity of the processes that generate them, but resting fundamentally on the projection of past trends. The projection of population density, for example, takes account of the fact that rates of growth of population varies greatly from state to state, the projection of per capita disposable income takes account of the entry of women into the labor force, and the projection of primary care physicians takes account of the shift from general practice to primary care specialties such as internal medicine and pediatrics. The effect of insurance is incorporated into the projections by means of several assumptions about the extent of coverage to be provided by National Health Insurance.

Feldstein's demand equation must be combined with a hospital bed supply equation if an equilibrating price is to be calculated.[1] For a given level of demand, the equilibrium price will be higher if there are fewer beds and lower if there are more beds. From 1963 to 1971, all short-term hospitals increased the number of beds per capita just enough to keep prices about one percent below what they would otherwise have been. Non-federal long-term hospitals allowed per capita beds to decline and raised prices about one percent above what they would otherwise have been. Our projections assume that past price-moderating behavior will be followed in the future and that in each class of hospitals (non-federal psychiatric, non-federal long-term, non-federal tuberculosis, federal, non-government non-profit short-term, for-profit short-term, and state and local short-term), per capita beds would continue to increase or decrease so as to affect rates of price increase, either by moderating or exacerbating them, just as in the past. This assumption differs only trivially in its effect on the projections of demand for administrators from assuming that the number of beds per capita will not change.

Table 1 illustrates the forecasts of expense per patient day for non-governmental, non-profit, short-term hospitals under four different assumptions about the level of National Health Insurance. These four assumptions are as follows. Without National Health Insurance, it is assumed that existing insurance plans remain in effect and that in 1975 the average patient pays about 10 percent of his hospital bill. National Health Insurance is assumed not to alter hospital coverage significantly for most people, but to extend to those who are presently unprotected or else inadequately protected more or less the same protection most of us have. Under assumptions A, B, and C, we assume that N.H.I. reduces the average payment from $.10 per dollar to $.09, $.08, and $.07 respectively. Further reduction weakens price as a restraint in the use of hospitals, and the equilibrating level of price is so high as to guarantee direct intervention in the form of some sort of rationing of service by the government. We have not considered the extreme case.

TABLE 1
PREDICTED EXPENSE PER PATIENT-DAY IN NGNPS HOSPITALS, 1975–1990
(1974 dollars)

National Health Insurance	Year			
	1975	1980	1985	1990
None	$157	$234	$322	$443
A	168	258	368	491
B	183	287	414	552
C	200	325	472	613

The Effect of H.M.O.'s

Expense per patient day could be moderated by a program of increasing the number of beds. But this is not the only way, short of rationing, that the demand pressure on hospital costs could be relieved. Experience with health maintenance organizations suggests that members are hospitalized less than comparable populations with ordinary hospital and health insurance coverage. The exact reason for the observed difference is not known, but it seems to be a real difference nevertheless. This means that hospital costs could be somewhat restrained by a successful program of H.M.O. This, in turn, would shift the demand for hospital administrators. To trace this effect we assumed establishment of an H.M.O. plan in 1974 under which H.M.O. formation would go on at a rate such that by 1978, 25 percent of the population of the United States would be enrolled. The rest of the population has conventional coverage, and after 1978 the proportion covered by H.M.O.'s remains at 25 percent, with enrollment growing only as fast as population. We assume that H.M.O. members use the hospital 30 percent less than comparable non-members. The effect of this program on hospital costs would be a reduction of about 10 percent in the costs given in Table 1 for all years except 1975.

Demand Projections for Hospital Administrators

Starting from a base of about 16,500 hospital administrators in 1971, we project a total of about 20,000 by 1990 regardless of N.H.I. levels of coverage. The principal effect of coverage level will be to shift the distribution of educational qualifications demanded by hospitals. In 1971, 45 percent of hospital administrators had a B.A. degree or less, while 55 percent had an M.A. degree or more. By 1990 these proportions would have shifted to about 10 percent and 90 percent even if N.H.I. is not established. If N.H.I. reduces the patient's payment to $.08 per dollar, these proportions will be about 5 percent and 95 percent. Even more striking will be the effect on the demand for administrators with Ph.D. or M.D. degrees. Fewer than 1 percent of the hospital administrators in our sample now hold such degrees. Our projection for 1990 is that about 8 percent will hold such degrees in the absence of N.H.I., and with N.H.I. paying all but $.08 on the dollar, the proportion will rise to almost 15 percent. We also project a shift toward specialized health administration training. About 40 percent now have such training. We project about 65 percent in 1990 without N.H.I., and about 75 percent with N.H.I.

The H.M.O. affects the training of administrators, but not their numbers. The magnitude of the effect is, however, small except for the case of the demand for Ph.D.-M.D. trained administrators. Under the H.M.O. plan and with N.H.I., the demand for such highly trained administrators would be about 10 percent in 1990 instead of 15 percent.

Conclusions

The demand for hospital administrators is projected to grow at a rate of about 1 percent per year through 1990. Not all components of this market will grow so slowly however. The number of administrators with M.D. and Ph.D. degrees will increase about 30-fold from the present small number of about 100. Even this change is well within the capacity of the present educational system. No special stimulation or encouragement is needed.

The principal reason for this finding, which seems counter to the experience of the past forty years, is that private hospital insurance has reached such a large fraction of the population and covers such a large part of the cost of hospitalization already, that even the introduction of an N.H.I. plan that provides generous coverage to the whole population will do little to further stimulate the demand for hospitalization.

NOTES

1. Martin S. Feldstein. "Hospital Cost Inflation: A Study of Nonprofit Price Dynamics." *American Economic Review,* LXI, 5, December, 1971. pp. 853–872.

Part II

A Report of
Commission Research

Authors in Part II

Charles J. Austin, Ph.D.
Presently Dean of Graduate Studies
  Trinity University, San Antonio
On leave from Xavier University
  Graduate Program in Hospital and
  Health Administration during study

James A. Ball, M.H.A.
Assistant Administrator and
  Director of Medical Services
  St. Anthony Hospital System
  Denver, Colorado
Assistant Administrator
  McKinley General Hospital
  Gallup, New Mexico

Daniel A. Clark, M.H.A.
Presently Assistant Director of the
  Kentucky January Program
  College of Allied Health Professions
  University of Kentucky
Administrative Resident at AUPHA
  during the study

Education for Health Administration: A Statistical Profile*

Background

The early roots of formal education for health administration can be traced to two sources: administrative courses offered by professional schools of public health and graduate programs designed to prepare students for careers in hospital administration.

The first three schools of public health in the United States were established in the early 1900s at Harvard, Yale, and Johns Hopkins Universities. The original focus of administrative education in these schools was on organization of community health services in official public health agencies with emphasis on the training of physicians who wished to become health officers in state and local agencies. Curriculum emphases focused on epidemiology, vital statistics, and the organization of preventive and environmental health services in a community. Many of the programs in public health administration still retain this focus.

For several years, schools of public health scrupulously avoided the more controversial subject of medical care administration which concentrated on organized methods for the delivery of personal health services. The first break in this tradition occurred during the 1930s with courses developed at the University of Michigan (Dr. Nathan Sinai) and Yale University (Dr. Franz Goldman). From these early beginnings, courses in medical care organization have flourished and are now offered in all schools of public health. Several of the schools also offer separate master's degree concentrations in medical care. The curricula of the medical programs focus broadly on the social, economic, and political factors which influence the organization of

---

* by Charles J. Austin, Daniel A. Clark, and James A. Ball.

personal health services. Students in the medical care programs have increasingly been drawn from individuals with a variety of backgrounds not limited to those with previous training in the health professions.

The first successful degree granting program in hospital administration was established at the University of Chicago in 1934 (there were a few earlier but abortive efforts). By the early 1950s 12 universities were offering degrees in this field. They focused on internal institutional management, and were closely connected to hospital administration practice through the use of local administrators as part-time faculty and the requirement for a nine to twelve month's administrative residency in a hospital following a period of academic work. The development of the programs during the 1950s and early 1960s was heavily influenced by the recommendations of the Commission on University Education in Hospital Administration.[1]

During the late 1960s, several new programs in hospital administration were established, and curriculum focus has gradually changed from concentration on running an institution to planning, organizing, and supervising the delivery of personal health services in concert with the larger community health system. Most of the programs have changed their names from hospital administration to "health services administration" or something comparable, and in 1973 the Association of University Programs in *Hospital* Administration became the Association of University Programs in *Health* Administration. About half of the programs have now adopted a two-year academic format with a summer externship replacing the year-long administrative residency.

As a result of federal legislation passed in 1966 (PL 89–749, Section 314), 25 universities established degree programs in comprehensive health planning in support of a new emphasis on voluntary health planning at the state and local level. Most of these planning programs were located in departments of schools offering health administration degrees, but others were freestanding without such affiliation. Their curriculum emphases range from planning as an administrative specialty to city planning to community organization and social planning.

Recent interest in health administration education at the graduate level has also been observed in schools of public administration which have recognized the growing convergence of health care and public policy. Additionally, schools of social work have developed an interest in health administration as a subspecialty of the developing field of human service administration .

Another important development in the field of health administration education is the recent emergence of undergraduate programs in health administration. Most of these programs are fewer than five years old, and they are located in both two-year community colleges and baccalaureate institutions. Although there have been several different approaches to the development of curricula at the undergraduate level, the majority of the programs state their objectives as preparation of graduates for middle-management positions in health institutions and agencies. However, some of the baccalaureate programs have objectives which are much closer to the future-executive orientation of graduate programs, and others focus on specialized areas of application, particularly long term care administration.

Survey Methodology

In order to build a demographic profile of this educational specialty field, the Commission conducted a series of questionnaire surveys in the spring and summer of 1973. Two of the questionnaires were designed to describe institutional activity on the graduate and undergraduate level. The remaining three surveys were designed to solicit the opinions of students, alumni, and employers about the quality of graduate education for health administration.

After pre-testing and revision, a 54-question survey instrument was mailed to 31 operational undergraduate programs in the fall of 1973. "Operational" was defined as an academic program having students enrolled during academic year 1972–73. (See Table 1.)

There existed at that time no central source of information about the location of undergraduate programs. The 31 that were surveyed resulted from inquiries made to the Association of University Programs in Health Administration, from examination of government publications, and from data supplied by Meharry University which had been attempting to organize undergraduate programs in this field. Eighteen completed questionnaires were returned, a response rate of 67 percent. (Four additional questionnaires were returned incomplete from universities whose programs were not yet operational.)

A questionnaire consisting of 82 questions was also sent to 72 operational graduate programs in health administration in the U.S. and Canada. The programs were identified through a series of inquiries to educational associations concerned with education for health administration including: the Association of University Programs in Health Administration, the Association of Schools of Public Health, the Association of Collegiate Schools of Business, and the National Association of Schools of Public Affairs and Administration. Of 67 U.S.

TABLE I
RESPONSES TO INSTITUTIONAL QUESTIONNAIRES

	Graduate			Under-Graduate
	U.S.	Canadian	Total	
Questionnaires mailed	67*	5	72	27**
Questionnaires returned	49	5	54	18
Response rate	73%	100%	75%	67%

* Seventy-one questionnaires were actually mailed, but eight respondents combined their answers into four responses.

** Thirty-one questionnaires were actually mailed but four were found not to be operational.

programs surveyed, 49 responded, (a response rate of 73 percent) and all five Canadian programs responded. The institutional survey instruments were designed to obtain descriptive information about educational activity. Due to constraints of time and resources, the Commission was unable to undertake an in-depth analysis of the quality of educational processes carried on within the institutions.

The response of the graduate programs by type of program was uneven, and the results may be biased accordingly. Ninety-four percent of the programs in hospital administration responded, 73 percent of the public health and medical care administration programs in schools of public health responded, and only 37 percent of the remainder (independent health planning programs, programs in public administration, etc.) responded to the questionnaire.

Concurrent with the institutional surveys, an additional study was developed to obtain value judgments from the "consumers" of graduate education in health administration. Separate but similar survey instruments were prepared for: students enrolled in their final year of study; 1971 graduates; and employers of the 1971 graduates. Names and addresses were obtained through an inquiry to all of the 72 graduate programs mentioned above. At the time of the survey, there were very few alumni from undergraduate programs in health administration, and hence the survey was limited to graduate programs. Table II gives a capsule summary of the response patterns to these surveys.

Major Findings

1. Educational programs in health administration are located in a wide variety of settings within their parent colleges and universities,

TABLE II
Responses to Student, Graduate, Employer Survey Questionnaire by Category of Graduate Program

Category of Program	Students	Graduates	Employers
Total Questionnaires Mailed To:			
Hospital administration	1,011	580	
— Returned	615	291	
— Response rate	61%	50%	
Medical care administration	52	29	
— Returned	22	13	
— Response rate	42%	45%	
Comprehensive health planning	100	85	
— Returned	36	36	
— Response rate	36%	42%	
Public health administration	293	213	
— Returned	133	82	
— Response rate	45%	38%	
Total Questionnaires Mailed	1,456	907	907
Total Returned	806	422	241
Response Rate	55%	47%	27%

and specific organizational locus seems much less important than does access to university-wide resources.

2. The number of graduate programs has more than doubled in the last ten years. The baccalaureate programs have only recently opened their doors. The oldest undergraduate program graduated its first class in 1966. There appears to be a continuing growth trend in this field at both the graduate and undergraduate level.

3. The Commission has estimated that 2,100 degrees were awarded by U.S. graduate programs in academic year 1972–73. If the growth rate of programs continues, by 1980 over 3,000 graduate degrees will be awarded annually. This assumes a growth rate of 5 percent, a conservative figure when compared to growth in recent years.

4. Women are badly underrepresented among the student bodies of educational programs in health administration (23 percent of graduate students and 31 percent of the baccalaureate students). While some progress has been made in recruiting black students (10 percent of graduate students and 12 percent of baccalaureate students), very little progress has been made in bringing Chicanos and Native Americans into this field.

5. Although there is a high ratio of applicants to those accepted into graduate programs (4:1), the undergraduate academic preparation

of those who apply for graduate programs is only average with mean undergraduate grade point averages ranging from 2.5 to 3.3, and mean Graduate Record Exam scores ranging from 950 to 1260.

6. The total full-time faculty to student ratio is good (1:8), but the range is wide. Forty-eight percent of the respondent programs had faculties of four members or fewer. The predominance of small faculties limits the time available for research, continuing education, and community service.

7. Women are grossly underrepresented on faculties, comprising only about 15 percent of both graduate and undergraduate program faculties.

8. There is an overdependence on "soft" sources of funding, thus indicating inadequate backing by parent universities and a large degree of vulnerability to the vagaries of federal budgets and educational support policies. Graduate programs are more vulnerable then undergraduate programs.

9. From analysis of broad curricular subjects, the surveys disclosed little variance in approach to education for health administration between graduate and undergraduate levels, possibly indicating poor articulation between these levels.

10. Little relationship can be found between placement of graduates and availability of specialty tracks in the curricula.

11. There is a general agreement among students, graduates and employers about the relevance and emphasis of graduate program curriculum areas. Students and graduates tend to be more critical of their curricula than are employers. Deficiencies in graduate preparation seem to be in the areas of:

- Financial management,
- Understanding of medical and nursing practice,
- Personnel administration,
- Political science,
- Quantitative methods in administrative problem solving.

12. Employers are fairly well satisfied with the products of the graduate programs, 85 percent of those polled preferring graduates of health administration to fill their vacancies in administrative positions. (There is a definite bias here, however, since 66 percent of the employers themselves have master's level education and 23 percent also hold some type of doctoral degree.)

13. Ninety-four percent of the employers surveyed felt that the graduates of the programs were highly or moderately well-prepared

for entry level positions. Students and graduates were a bit more critical. Sixty-five percent of the students and 66 percent of the graduates rated the quality of their education to be satisfactory to above average.

14. There is general agreement by all parties surveyed (faculties, students, alumni, and employers) that:

- Undergraduate programs should be encouraged.
- Professional associations should require mandatory continuing education and/or examination as preferable to governmental licensure of health administrators.
- Minimum standards of educational quality should be established and programs should be evaluated from outside by accrediting agencies.

Analysis and Discussion

GRADUATE PROGRAMS

Graduate programs, almost equally divided between public (55 percent) and private (45 percent) universities, are found in a wide variety of settings within their parent universities. The most common locus, 22 of the 54 respondents, is the school of public health (Table III). An emerging trend is the development of formal interdisciplinary programs involving two or more colleges or professional schools.

There has been rapid growth in the number of programs within

TABLE III
ORGANIZATIONAL LOCUS OF PROGRAMS

Locus	U.S. No.	%	Canada No.	%	Total No.	%
Schools of Public Health	20	41%	2	40%	22	40%
Schools of Medicine	5	10%	2	40%	7	13%
Schools of Business	4	8%	1	20%	5	9%
Schools of Public Administration	2	4%			2	4%
Schools of Business & Public Administration	4	8%			4	7%
Schools of Allied Health	4	8%			4	7%
Independent	4	8%			4	7%
Interdisciplinary	5	10%			5	9%
Other	1	2%			1	2%

the last five to ten years; 31 percent of the reporting programs are less than five years old and 55 percent are less than ten years old.

Table IV presents student enrollment data. Though the programs average 46 full-time and 11 part-time students, the range of class size is broad (0 to 279 full-time students and 0 to 178 part-time students). In general, the students are mature, the average age being 28 years, and predominantly male.

Minority students, particularly Chicanos and Native Americans, are underrepresented on student bodies. There are also needs for increased efforts to recruit female students. Only 23 percent of the student population of U.S. graduate programs are women.

The ratio of students applying to entering the programs is relatively

TABLE IV
STUDENT ENROLLMENT IN PROGRAMS

Student Body	U.S.	Canada
	n=48	n=5
1. Total Students Enrolled — 1972–73	2,785 (3,900)*	179
2. Breakdown		
Average number of full-time students per program	46	33
— Range	0–279	7–50
Average number of part-time students per program	11	3
— Range	0–178	0–9
% Male students	77%	68%
% Female students	23%	32%
Minority:		
% Black students	10%	
% Spanish American	2%	
% Native American	0.7%	
3. Median Age of Students	28	30
— Range	23–36	24–40
4. Ratio of Students Applying to Entering	4:1	5:1
5. Entering Academic Credentials		
— Range of Mean Graduate Record Exam Scores	950 to 1260	
— Range of Mean Undergraduate Grade Point Averages	2.5 to 3.3	

* Projection to entire population.

high (4:1) suggesting a trend toward multiple applications by students to several programs. Academic credentials prior to admission to the programs reflect only average quality. Further, once a student enters a program, there is little chance he will not complete his requirements for a degree. Ninety-three percent of U.S. students and 90 percent of Canadian students complete the program and receive a degree.

Table V presents data on placement of graduates of the master's degree programs in health administration.

TABLE V
NUMBER OF GRADUATES OF HEALTH ADMINISTRATION PROGRAMS

	U.S.	Canada
	n=41	n=5
Total number of graduates through 1972–73	10,000 (15,000)*	1,568
Total number of degrees awarded in 1972–73	1,278 (2,100)*	85
Most common placement of graduates (% of all graduates reported)		
— Hospital administration	53%	41%
— Government health agency	13%	35%
— Comprehensive health planning	5%	5%
— Unknown—not in health care	11%	8%
(All other categories less than 5%)		

* Projected to entire U.S. population (67 programs)

Graduates tend to be placed primarily in hospitals with hospital administration, government agency administration, and health planning collectively accounting for over 70 percent of the total placements reported. Very few graduates took positions in mental health, ambulatory care, or long term care administration even though 24, 22, and 10 percent of the programs respectively stated that they offer specialty tracks in these fields. Additionally, fewer than 2 percent of the graduates took positions in third-party reimbursement organizations or in voluntary health agencies.

The faculty of graduate programs are generally male (87 percent) and 61 percent hold the doctoral degree. There is a quite favorable faculty to student ratio (1:8). In the U.S. the average number of full-time faculty per program is 5.8 and the average number of part-time faculty is 8.5 These figures are mitigated, however, by a rather large range in distribution of faculty in the programs. The 44 respondents to this survey question listed as full-time faculty a range from one to 18 teachers. Fully 48 percent of the programs, however, report four faculty members or fewer. These data imply that most faculties are quite small, some lacking the critical mass necessary to carry out a comprehensive program of teaching, continuing education, research and community service.

One unexpected finding of the survey was the similarity of response to questions concerning curriculum content. Almost every program listed the following as content areas: administrative and organizational theory, medical care organization, hospital administration, health economics, and electronic data processing. In most cases, these courses are required and an interdisciplinary approach is followed.

In a survey of student, alumni, and employer views of the educational process (to be discussed later in this chapter), respondents were asked to evaluate strengths and deficiencies in curriculum content areas. All three groups of respondents agreed that financial management, medical and nursing practice, personnel administration, political science, and quantitative methods were the greatest weaknesses of the programs. Further study of the curriculum content of the graduate programs tends to explain these deficiencies. The data suggest that, in many cases, the above courses are taught by program faculty members rather than by specialists in these fields from other departments of the university. (see Table VI) This suggests that there are needs to strengthen interdisciplinary ties for instruction in these specialty content areas.

TABLE VI
Content Areas and Program Treatment*

Content Areas	Times Mentioned	Required Courses		Elective Courses	
		Program Faculty	Interdisciplinary	Program Faculty	Interdisciplinary
Administrative and Organization Theory	48	26	17	11	7
Medical Care Organization	46	34	6	8	5
Electronic Data Processing	43	15	15	8	16
Health Economics	43	28	5	11	12
Hospital Administration	43	34	1	9	4
Financial Management	42	29	10	11	10
Health Planning	41	25	1	16	5

* U.S. Programs. N=48

Table VII presents data on activities of the faculty other than graduate student instruction. Program faculty report that, on the average, 9 percent of their time is spent on continuing education. Again, there is a wide range of response from 0 percent to 51 percent of faculty time. Almost all activity in this area is devoted to health administration practitioners, as opposed to consumers, board members, and others involved in health policy and administration.

TABLE VII
Non-Teaching Activities of Graduate Program Faculty

Activities	U.S.	Canada
a. Average % of faculty time devoted to continuing education	8.8%	7.0%
— Range	0–51%	0–15%
b. Average % of program budget devoted to continuing education	4%	6%
c. Average % of faculty time devoted to research	21%	18%
— Range	0–60%	5–40%
d. Average % of program budget devoted to research*	26%	31%

* Five programs accounted for over 50% of the total research dollars reported in the survey.

Much more non-teaching faculty time is devoted to research. Programs report an average of 21 percent of their faculty time in this area. (This percentage ranges from 0 percent to 60 percent.) However, five of the 48 reporting U.S. programs account for over 50 percent of the research being carried out.

Forty-five U.S. and Canadian programs answered budgetary questions in the survey. Total budgets ranged from $52,000 to $1,438,000 per year. Teaching budgets ranged from $42,000 to $550,000. Table VIII presents a frequency distribution of the size of program budgets.

Fifty of the graduate programs answered a non-structured question concerning program objectives. Those objectives mentioned most often (26 percent of the programs) concerned manpower and curriculum, and indicated that the programs view their role as preparation of generalist administrators for the field.

Several programs mentioned modification of student values toward the role of health in a community setting or toward a humanistic philosophy as a major objective (10 programs). Community service

TABLE VIII
Frequency Distribution of Program Budgets

Total Budget* (Thousands)	U.S. n=41	Canada n=4
0–100	6	—
101–200	10	2
201–300	4	—
301–400	4	1
401–500	4	1
501–600	3	—
601–700	—	—
701–800	2	—
801–900	2	—
901–1000	2	—
$ 1001–Over	4	—

* Fully 70 percent of these funds come from federal grants and contracts and private foundation grants, thus indicating a precarious over-reliance on "soft" sources of funding.

objectives revolved around technical assistance to health institutions and agencies (11 programs), while six programs mentioned the provision of educational services for the community as an objective.

Forty-two of the 54 respondents answered another open-ended question concerning educational myths. Analysis of the responses brings to light many controversies and disagreements among educators over issues which have lingered since professional education was first conceived. Very little consensus could be gleaned from the data. However, there seemed to be some feeling that there is no necessary relationship between graduate education and a student's future success (12 programs stressed this point). In all other issues, from the value of theory over practice to the value of practitioner input to the value of the residency requirement, the programs reached overwhelming agreement—to disagree.

Undergraduate Programs

Undergraduate programs are found in both public and private institutions in fairly equal proportions. Sixty percent of the associate degree respondents (three programs) and 62 percent of the baccalaureate respondents (eight programs) are found in public institutions with the remainder in private settings. Programs are located in a wide variety of settings within the parent school with Business Administration and Allied Health being most common.

The majority of the baccalaureate programs offer a Bachelor of Science degree with health administration as a single major field of study. Undergraduate education in this field is rather new, with no responding program over ten years of age.

The composition of the student body of undergraduate programs is shown in Table IX.

TABLE IX

COMPOSITION OF STUDENT BODY OF UNDERGRADUATE HEALTH ADMINISTRATION PROGRAMS, ACADEMIC YEAR, 1972–73

Student Body Categories	Associate Programs n=5	Baccalaureate Programs n=12
Total number of students enrolled	86	491
Breakdowns: Full-time students	51%	97%
Part-time students	49%	3%
Male students	57%	69%
Female students	43%	31%
Minority Groups: Black	2%	12%
Spanish Surname	5%	3%
Native American	0%	(less than 1%)
Age distribution: Under 25 years of age	40%	73%
25 to 35 years of age	40%	22%
Over 35 years of age	20%	5%

The student bodies of undergraduate programs are younger than those of the graduate programs as would be expected, and they contain a slightly higher percentage of women than do the graduate programs, thus confirming a finding of the Carnegie Commission on Higher Education that the proportion of women enrolled decreases as the education level increases.[2] The percentage of black students in the four-year programs approximately equates that of blacks in the general population but the same is not true for the associate degree programs. Undergraduate programs were reluctant to provide data on admission test scores of entering students, but the small amount of data that were available indicate about average performance on these tests in comparison with other students entering the parent institution.

Although there are not much data as yet on placement of graduates from two-year and four-year undergraduate programs, the trend appears toward long term care administration for associate degree graduates and hospital administration for baccalaureate graduates. Thirteen percent of the 1972–73 baccalaureate graduates were continuing on to graduate study in health administration. See Table X.

TABLE X
Graduates and Placements in Undergraduate Health Administration Programs

Graduates and Placements	Associate Degree Programs n=4	Baccalaureate Programs* n=12
Total number of graduates through 1972–73	32	405
Total number of degrees awarded in 1972–73	13	170
Most common placement of graduates (% of all graduates):		
— Hospital administration	22%	50%
— Long term care administration	78%	5%
— Comprehensive health planning agencies	—	10%
— Continued on to graduate school:		
— In health administration	—	13%
— In other fields of study	—	9%

* All other categories less than 5% each.

As shown by Table XI, faculties of the undergraduate programs are smaller than those of graduate programs. Only about one-third of the full-time faculty members of the baccalaureate programs hold the doctoral degree. As with graduate programs, the faculties are predominantly male.

TABLE XI
Profile of Faculties of Undergraduate Programs in Health Administration

Faculties of Undergraduate Programs	Associate Degree Programs	Baccalaureate Programs
a. Average number of full-time faculty per program	1.6	2.8
Average number of part-time faculty per program	3.0	3.3
b. Male faculty members	78%	85%
Female faculty members	22%	15%
c. Proportion of full-time faculty holding doctoral degrees	14%	37%

The results of the survey of non-teaching activities of the faculties are shown in Table XII.

Non-teaching activity indicates some differences from graduate programs. Undergraduate programs have higher involvement in con-

TABLE XII
Non-Teaching Activities in Undergraduate Programs in Health Administration

Non-teaching Activities	Associate Degree Programs	Baccalaureate Programs
a. Number of programs involved in some form of continuing education activities	3	8
b. Number of programs involved in some form of research	1	7
c. Number of programs involved in formal service programs to community agencies and organizations	—	8

tinuing education with three of the associate degree and eight of the baccalaureate programs so involved. These eleven programs carried out 24 courses in the last two years, primarily oriented to practicing health administrators.

Table XIII surveys the curricular structure of undergraduate programs. Approximately 25 percent of the curricula of undergraduate programs are devoted to specific courses in health administration, the remainder to related courses and general education subjects. In examining some of the specific course offerings listed on the individual questionnaires, there is evident a high degree of overlap between the curricula of graduate and undergraduate programs, and also between two-year and four-year programs.

Table XIV presents budgetary data for the undergraduate programs. Although the average teaching budget is close to $100,000, one-half of the respondents reported teaching budgets under $50,000.

As with the graduate programs, "soft" sources of funding have become the backbone of baccalaureate program financing with 55 percent of the bachelor's level budgets financed through federal grants and contracts.

One of the more interesting responses from the undergraduate survey concerned the stated reasons for starting an undergraduate program in health administration. A majority of the respondents stated needs to fill manpower shortages in their specific community or region and to develop a new breed of administrator. However, manpower needs did not appear to have been systematically examined by most of the programs.

In contrast to graduate programs, undergraduate objectives are decidedly goal oriented and practical in approach. In stating objectives,

TABLE XIII
Curricula of Undergraduate Programs in Health Administration

Curricula	Associate Degree Programs	Baccalaureate Programs
	n=5	n=13
a. Overall structure (% of total curriculum)		
— Health administration courses	22%	24%
— Courses directly related to health administration	32%	30%
— General education courses	46%	46%
b. Number of programs with specialties: Functional specialty tracks in:		
— Financial management	1	3
— Planning	1	4
— Personnel administration	1	3
— Systems analysis	—	2
Organizational or Programmatic specialties:		
— Hospital administration	—	5
— Public health administration	—	3
— Mental health administration	—	2
— Ambulatory care administration	—	4
— Long term care administration	2	3
c. Experiential components of the curriculum: Number of the programs with:		
— Residency of 0 to 3 months duration	2	6
— Residency of 4 to 6 months duration	—	2
— Continuous part-time field work concurrent with on-campus study	3	3

only three of the 13 programs made specific reference to instilling philosophical values about health care delivery.

The majority of the programs list the preparation of middle management personnel as a major objective (85 percent). Other objectives include: (a) preparation for graduate education (46 percent); (b) diversity in type of administration or job market preparation (38 percent); (c) minority recruitment and preparation (23 percent); (d) preparation for specific populations or regions (31 percent).

Associate degree programs can be characterized from their objectives as training sites for middle management in hospitals (25 percent) or administrators or assistants in long term care institutions (50 percent). The emphasis tends to be on the immediate and practical, exemplified by outside field experience, for immediate entry on the job market.

TABLE XIV
Financing of Undergraduate Programs in Health Administration

Average Annual Budget for Programs	Associate Degree Programs $n=3$	Baccalaureate Programs[a] $n=10$
For teaching	$ 11,400	$ 97,362[b]
— Range	$5,000–15,000	$13,000–328,332
For student support	$ 333	$ 32,348[c]
— Range	$ 0–1,000	$ 0–202,500
For research	$ 666	$ 12,160[d]
— Range	$ 0–2,000	$ 0–100,000
For continuing education	$ 5,000	$ 10,420[e]
— Range	$ 0–2,000	$ 0–100,000
Other	$ 3,000	$ 21,766
— Range	$ 0–5,000	$ 0–118,854
TOTAL	$ 20,399	$ 173,756[f]
— Range	$5,000–32,000	$18,500–400,000
Source of Funding (% of budget)		
— Federal Grants		55%
— State Government		30%
— Foundations		3%
— Internal University Funds	100%	10%
— Other		2%

[a] Does not include the Navy-GWU program. Their total budget is funded through the Department of the Navy.
[b] Five of the ten respondents had teaching budgets less than $50,000.
[c] Four programs had no student support funds.
[d] Six programs had no research funds.
[e] Seven programs had no continuing education funds.
[f] Four programs had budgets under $100,000.

Surveys of Students, Graduates, and Employers

As mentioned earlier, the Commission attempted to gain some measure of the quality of education by questioning the "consumer" of educational services. Students and graduates could evaluate the process of education, and employers could evaluate its output.

One of the most important and informative areas of these surveys concerned the adequacy of curriculum content areas. The student and graduate groups were asked to rate specific content areas according to their relevance and degree of emphasis in the curriculum. Employers were asked to rate the content areas according to the degree of importance to the job which the graduate filled as well as the degree to which the graduate was prepared to carry out entry-level responsibilities.

For the most part, employers' responses were uniform for both requirement and qualification ratings. Where a particular content area is heavily required by the job, the graduate is rated as well qualified. The two major exceptions to this were personnel administration and financial management. Both of these areas were rated high in importance but graduates were only moderately well qualified.

Graduates were more critical in their ratings. They complained that many content areas, though relevant, are not adequately emphasized in curricula. Most notable in this category are political science, computer applications, personnel administration, financial management, and medical-nursing practice.

Students were the most zealous in their rating. Nearly every content area was rated higher in relevance than the graduate's, but the same pattern emerges. There is a large discrepancy between relevance and curriculum emphasis in political science, medical sociology, health law, industrial relations, computer applications, personnel administration, financial management, and understanding of medical-nursing practice.

In addition to rating curricula by content area, each group was asked to rank the strongest and weakest areas (employers were asked to list the most crucial and most deficient areas). Again the results are quite uniform. Administrative and organizational theory, medical care organization, and comprehensive health planning were agreed to be the strongest and among the most important. Employers indicated that the most crucial areas are also the most deficient, particularly financial management, personnel administration, research methodology, and understanding of medical-nursing practice. Table XV shows the results of this analysis.

Both students and graduates were asked to grade the overall quality of their educational experience. The modal evaluation for both groups was "above average." (see Table XVI)

Both students and graduates responded similarly to questions regarding value of the residency field experience. On the whole, the field experience was rated high in value. (see Table XVII)

Most students and graduates reported little or no difficulty in finding jobs. There was no significant difference in graduates' responses by

TABLE XV
Employers' Perceptions of the Most Crucial and Most Deficient Curriculum Content Areas in Regard to Job Performance

Most Crucial	Most Deficient
1. Administrative and Organizational Theory	1. Financial Management
2. Medical Care Organization	2. Personnel Administration
3. Financial Management	3. Research Methodology
4. Personnel Administration	4. Medical/Nursing Practice
5. Research Methodology	5. Quantitative Techniques
6. Comprehensive Health Planning	6. Political Science/Government Relations
7. Medical/Nursing Practice	7. Systems Analysis/E.D.P.

Students and Graduates Perceptions of Strongest and Weakest Curriculum Content Areas

Strongest Content Areas	Weakest Content Areas
1. Administrative and Organizational Theory (General)	1. Financial Management
2. Administrative and Organizational Theory (Health Specific)	2. Systems Analysis/E.D.P.
3. Medical Care Organization	3. Personnel Administration
4. Comprehensive Health Planning	4. Health Law
5. Applied Statistics	

TABLE XVI
Overall Evaluation of Educational Programs

Evaluation	Students	Graduates
Needs improvement	20%	18%
Satisfactory	26%	23%
Above average	38%	43%
Superior	16%	16%

sex. (Members of religious communities were excluded from the analysis when sex was used as a controlling variable.)

Ninety-four percent of the employers rated the graduates highly or moderately well prepared. There was also strong agreement that the graduate was better prepared than an individual with no such training.

TABLE XVII
EVALUATION OF FIELD EXPERIENCE COMPONENT OF CURRICULUM

Evaluation of Field Experience	Students	Graduates
Very valuable—the most important part of my program	44%	32%
Valuable—of equal importance to academic work	43%	45%
Of some value but less important than academic work	10%	18%
Of minimum value	3%	5%

Sixty-three percent of the respondents, however, reported that they do have administrative personnel at approximately the same level of responsibility who have not had formal education in health administration or planning. Eighty-six percent of the respondents prefer a health administration or planning program graduate when vacancies do occur.

There is rather strong agreement among students, graduates, and administrators that subject specialization is desirable. Much less agreement is evident when the question of institutional specialization is approached. Though small majorities of students and graduates (55.1 percent and 51.6 percent respectively) saw a need for such specialization, a majority of employers disagreed. Table XVIII presents the relative frequency of response as to which subject specialties should be offered.

OPINIONS AND PRIORITIES

A set of parallel questions was asked all the groups surveyed about: (1) priorities for input into educational objectives and policies; (2) priorities for activities other than entry-level education for health programs; and (3) opinions on certain key issues in health adminis-

TABLE XVIII
PERCENTAGE OF STUDENTS, GRADUATES, AND EMPLOYERS WHO FAVOR SUBJECT SPECIALIZATION IN THE CURRICULA

Specialty Area	Students	Graduates	Employers
1. Financial management	49.2%	41.8%	47.7%
2. Planning	59.1%	52.2%	54.8%
3. Personnel administration	31.3%	28.0%	41.5%
4. Communications	16.6%	17.5%	22.4%
5. Systems Analysis	40.8%	34.7%	39.4%
6. Policy Analysis	23.7%	20.9%	25.3%

tration education. For the most part, the responses were predictable, reflecting the interests of the different groups involved. A detailed display of the results are included in Tables XIX and XX to follow.

The first question attempted to delineate who should be involved in formulating objectives and policy for educational programs. The consumers of the programs (students, graduates and employers) placed high priority on practitioner input, and faculty members tended to assign high priority to their own input as well as that of practitioners and students. Those on the periphery of the programs (health professionals in the community, consumer representatives, etc.) were not viewed as important sources of input into the educational policy process.

TABLE XIX
PRIORITIES FOR INPUT INTO EDUCATIONAL OBJECTIVES AND POLICIES
(Rank Order)

Input By:	U.S. Graduate Programs	U.S. Undergrad. Programs	Students	Employers	Alumni
Practicing Administrators in the Community	2	1	1	1	1
Faculty	1	2	2	2	2
Alumni	5	7	3	4	3
Health Professionals in the Community	4	3	4	3	4
Students	3	4	5	5	5
Consumers	6	5	6	6	6
Other	7	6	7	7	7

The questionnaire also listed a series of activities in addition to entry-level teaching thought to be appropriate for educational programs in health administration. The surveyed groups were asked to assign priorities to these activities considering the limited resources most programs have at hand. There is considerable variance in response patterns, but again the consumers formed a fairly united front. Students, graduates, employers, and undergraduate programs felt continuing education of alumni and practitioners to be of highest priority. The undergraduate response is understandable in light of their often stated objectives and activities concerning continuing education. Graduate programs differ markedly from other respondents in the priority given to continuing education. These programs seem to be more

TABLE XX
Priorities for Activities Other than Entry-Level Teaching
(Rank Order)

Activities	U.S. Graduate Programs	U.S. Undergrad. Programs	Students	Employers	Alumni
Continuing education of program graduates	5	2	1	1	1
Continuing education of practicing administrators in the community	3	1	2	2	2
Research	1	4	3	3	3
Technical assistance	2	3	4	4	4
Public policy formulation	4	4	5	6	5
Special education for Board Members	6	6	6	5	6
Special education for consumers	7	7	7	7	7
Special education for others	8	5	8	8	8

interested in research and technical assistance programs, an understandable position in light of the current faculty reward system. One other tendency for all groups is to delegate "community education," continuing education for board members, consumers and others, to the lowest priority.

All respondents were asked whether educational programs should be concerned primarily with entry level preparation rather than taking a future executive approach. Associate degree programs strongly agreed and baccalaureate programs also agreed, but not as strongly. Students, alumni, and faculty of the graduate programs all disagreed but employers were ambivalent about the question.

Responses to the remaining opinion questions were fairly uniform across groups. Students, graduates, baccalaureate, associate and graduate programs all agreed that continued development of undergraduate programs in health administration should be encouraged. (Employers were not asked this question.) All groups agreed that professional associations should require mandatory continuing education and/or exams for continued membership, in lieu of government licensure, which was strongly opposed. There was also uniform agreement with the establishment of minimum standards of quality and outside evaluation of educational programs by accrediting agencies. Finally, there was general agreement that the programs should attempt to alter the values of students.

Complete tabulations of all survey results are included in the Appendices which follow. Primary data have been retained by the Commission and will be available for further research by serious scholars upon request.

Notes

1. Commission on University Education in Hospital Administration. *University Education for Administration in Hospitals.* Washington, D.C.: American Council on Education, 1954.
2. Carnegie Commission on Higher Education. *Opportunities for Women in Higher Education.* New York: McGraw-Hill, October, 1973.

Appendices — Detailed Tabulations
Survey of Graduate Programs in Health Administration †

QUESTION 1 Type of parent institution of programs

	49 U.S. Programs	5 Canadian Programs
	%	%
Public ownership	55	80
Private ownership	45	20

QUESTION 3 Organizational locus of programs

	U.S. Programs		Canadian Programs	
	#	%*	#	%
School of Public Health	20	41	2	40
School of Medicine	5	10	2	40
School of Business Administration	4	8	1	20
School of Public Administration	2	4		
School of Allied Health	4	8		
School of Business & Public Administration	4	8		
Independent	4	8		
Interdisciplinary	5	10		
Other	1	2		
Total number of programs	49		5	

* Rounded figures

QUESTION 4 Kinds of master's degrees awarded

	U.S. Programs		Canadian Programs	
	#	%	#	%
MHA	12	18	3	60
MPH/MSPH	17	26	1	20
MBA	8	12		
MS	14	22	1	20
MA	3	5		
MPA	7	11		
Other	4	6		
Total number of programs	49		5	

† There is not a complete sequence of questions and answers given in this paper because some were open-ended questions which did not yield quantitative answers while others did not result in significant findings.

QUESTION 5 Age of programs

	U.S. #	U.S. %	Canadian #	Canadian %
0–5 years	15	31	1	25
6–10	12	24		
11–15	3	6	1	25
16–20	4	8		
Over 20	15	31	2	50
Total number of programs	49		4	

QUESTION 11 Student enrollment in programs

	48. U.S. Programs	5 Canadian Programs
Total Students Enrolled '72–'73	2,785 (3,900)*	179
Breakdown		
Average Full-Time	46	33
Range	0–279	7–50
Average Part-Time	11	3
Range	0–178	0–9
% Male Students	77%	68%
% Female Students	23%	32%
Minority:		
% Black Students	10%	
% Spanish American	2%	
% Native American	0.7%	

* Projection to entire population.

QUESTION 12 Median age of students in programs

	U.S.	Canadian
Median	28	30
Range	23–36	24–40

QUESTION 13 Students in programs — Highest previous degree*

	U.S. #	U.S. %	Canadian #	Canadian %
AB	738	32	23	17
BS	707	30	11	8
BBA	212	9	16	12
Other (or RN)	164	7	45	33
Total undergraduates	1,821	78	95	70
MA	64	3	6	4
MS	61	3	1	1
MBA	39	2	2	1
Other	94	4	0	00
Total masters	258	12	9	6
MD	172	7	32	24
DDS	44	2	0	00
PhD	12	.5	0	00
Other	18	.7	0	00
Total doctorates	246	10	32	24

* Percentages in rounded numbers.

QUESTION 14 Educational qualification of students in programs

	U.S.	Canadian
Undergraduate GPA (on 4.0 scale)		
Range	2.5–3.3	—
Number of Programs	39	—
Graduate Record Exam		
Range	950–1260	—
Number of Programs	25	—
Miller Analogy Exam		
Range	49–66	—
Number of Programs	7	—
ATGSB		
Range	450–602	—
Number of Programs	17	—

QUESTION 15 Students' work experience prior to entering program

	U.S.		Canadian	
	#	%	#	%
Full-Time Students				
Medical Practice	150	9	21	22
Nursing Practice	122	7	18	19
Health Administration	421	25	19	20
Other	469	28	10	11
Non-related	540	31	26	28
Total	1,702	100	94	100
Part-Time Students				
Medical Practice	18	5	1	10
Nursing Practice	42	10	4	40
Health Administration	189	48	5	50
Other	78	20	—	—
Non-related	69	17	—	—
Total	396	100	10	100

QUESTION 17 Elements of student admission criteria

	U.S. Programs		Canadian* Programs	
	#	%	#	%
Minimum Test Score				
Yes	22	46	—	—
No	26	54	—	—
Minimum GPA for Undergraduate Work				
Yes	36	73	5	83
No	13	27	1	17
Personal Interview with Faculty				
Yes	32	67	3	50
No	16	33	3	50
Letters of Reference				
Yes	45	94	2	40
No	3	06	3	60
Personal Interview with Alumni				
Yes	11	23	2	33
No	37	77	4	67

* Includes two reports from the University of Toronto—Diploma of Public Health and Diploma in Health Administration.

QUESTION 20 Ratio of students applying to entering

Ratio	4:1	5:1

QUESTION 21 Percentage of students who complete program and receive degree

	41 U.S. Programs	5 Canadian Programs
Average Percentage	93%	90%
Range	50–100%	75–98%

QUESTION 22 Number of full-time and part-time program faculty by rank and sex

	48 U.S. Programs		5 Canadian Programs	
RANK	No. of Male Faculty	No. of Female Faculty	No. of Male Faculty	No. of Female Faculty
Full Professor	61	2	8	0
Associate Professor, Tenured	28	1	4	3
Associate Professor, Not Tenured	30	7	4	0
Assistant Professor	85	10	7	3
Instructor	44	12	3	1
TOTAL FULL-TIME FACULTY	248	32	26	7
TOTAL PART-TIME FACULTY	353	56	22	2

Question 22 continued on next page.

FREQUENCY DISTRIBUTION — GRADUATE PROGRAM, FULL-TIME FACULTY*
(U.S. only)

Number of Faculty	Frequency
1	4
2	4
3	5
4	8
5	5
6	4
7	2
8	3
9	2
10	4
14	1
17	1
18	1
Total	44

* 48% of programs have four faculty or fewer.

Number of Faculty	Frequency	%	Cum. %
1–4	21	48	48
5–8	14	32	80
9–12	6	14	94
13–16	1	2	96
17–20	2	4	100
	44		

QUESTION 23   Highest degree held by program faculty members

	U.S.		Canadian	
	#	%	#	%
Full-Time Faculty				
PhD	91	33	10	31
MD/MPH	32	12	8	25
MD	14	5	3	9
Other doctorates	36	12	0	0
MPH	18	6	0	0
MHA	40	14	6	19
Other masters	54	18	5	16

QUESTION 24 Academic rank of program directors

	U.S. #	U.S. %	Canadian #	Canadian %
Full Professors	26	54	3	60
Associate Professors	19	40	1	20
Assistant Professors	2	4	1	20
Other	1	2	0	0

QUESTION 26 Use of funding *(in thousands)*

	41 U.S. Programs	4 Canadian Programs
Teaching—Mean	$164	$160
Range	42–550	78–277
Student Support—Mean	85	2
Range	0-567	0–8
Research—Mean	113	90
Range	0–1,121	0–157
Continuing Education—Mean	16	18
Range	0–139	0–59
Other (i.e., Administration)—Mean	55	16
Range	0–552	0–28
Total—Mean	$433	$286
Range	52–1,438	161–462

FREQUENCY DISTRIBUTION OF PROGRAM BUDGETS

Total Budget (Thousands)	41 U.S. Programs	4 Canadian Programs
$ 0–100	6	—
101–200	10	2
201–300	4	—
301–400	4	1
401–500	4	1
501–600	3	—
601–700	—	—
701–800	2	—
801–900	2	—
901–1000	2	—
1001–Over	4	—

QUESTION 27 Average financing of graduate programs in health administration

	U.S. $ Av. (%)	Canadian $ Av. (%)
Source of Funding (in thousands)		
Federal Grants and Contracts	273 (63%)	60 (21%)
Range	$0–1,142	$16-118
State and Local Government	37 (9%)	59 (20%)
Range	0–277	0–130
Private Foundations	32 (7%)	8 (3%)
Range	0–189	0–25
Internal University Funds	75 (17%)	159 (56%)
Range	0–281	87–306
Other	17 (4%)	0 (0%)
Range	0–254	

QUESTION 28 Effects of proposed cutbacks in federal funds

	U.S.	Canadian
Affected?		
Yes	34	N/A
No	13	
How Much? (in thousands)		
Student Aid	$2,811	N/A
Salaries	1,504	
Support Services	629	
Total	$4,944	

QUESTION 32 Comprehensive exams required to complete program

	U.S. Programs		Canadian Programs*	
	#	%	#	%
Yes	21	43	1	17
Written	8		0	
Oral	7		0	
Both	6		1	
No	28	57	5	83

* Includes two responses from University of Toronto—Diploma of Public Health and Diploma in Health Administration.

QUESTION 33 Master's thesis requirements

	U.S. Programs		Canadian Programs*	
	#	%	#	%
Required	19	39	3	50
Optional	16	33	2	33
Neither	14	28	1	17

* Includes two responses from University of Toronto—Diploma of Public Health and Diploma in Health Administration.

QUESTIONS 34 and 35 Content areas and program treatment in 48 U.S. programs

	Times Mentioned	Required		Elective	
		Program Faculty	Interdisciplinary	Program Faculty	Interdisciplinary
Administrative and Organization Theory	48	26	17	11	7
Medical Care Organization	46	34	6	8	5
Electronic Data Processing	43	15	15	8	16
Health Economics	43	28	5	11	12
Hospital Administration	43	34	1	9	4
Financial Management	42	29	10	11	10
Health Planning	41	25	1	16	5

QUESTION 36 Specialty tracks

	49 U.S. Programs		5 Canadian Programs	
	#	%	#	%
Functional Specialty Tracks				
Financial Management	16	33	1	20
Planning	23	47	1	20
Personnel Administration	10	20	0	0
Communications	3	6	0	0
Systems Analysis	16	33	1	20
Policy Analysis	12	24	1	20
Research	2	4	0	0
EDP	1	2	0	0
Law	4	8	0	0
Economics	1	2	0	0
Administrative Medicine	1	2	0	0
Labor Relations	1	2	0	0
Program Specialty Tracks				
Ambulatory Care Administration	11	22	1	20
Hospital Administration	25	51	3	60
Long Term Care Administration	5	10	0	0
Mental Health Administration	12	24	1	20
Public Health Administration	13	27	2	40

QUESTION 38 Experiential components of program curriculum

	49 U.S. Programs	5 Canadian Programs
Pre-admission Clerkship	4	—
Residency		
0–3 months	17	—
4–6 months	9	3
7–9 months	7	—
9–12 months	11	2
12 months or more	—	—
Concurrent Experience	18	—

QUESTION 39 Doctoral degree

	49 U.S. Programs		5 Canadian Programs	
	#	%	#	%
Yes	25	51	0	0
No	24	49	5	100
Major Fields of Concentration				
Health Administration	16			
Health Policy Administration	3			
Health Economics	3			
Research	5			
Health Planning	5			
Maternal and Child Health	1			
International Health	1			
Mental Health Administration	1			
Medical Care Organization	3			
Business w/Health Admin. Major	2			

QUESTION 40 Total number degrees granted by programs to date

	41 U.S.* Programs	5 Canadian Programs
Total	10,000	1,568
Average/Program	256	314

* Eight programs did not answer.

QUESTION 41 Degrees awarded 1972–73

	46 U.S. Programs	5 Canadian Programs
MHA	332	46
MPH/MSPH	557	14
MBA	111	—
MPA	57	—
MS	154	1
MA	49	—
Other	18	24
Total	1,278	85

QUESTION 42 Placement of program graduates*

	43 U.S. Programs	4 Canadian Programs
Hospital Administration	53%	41%
Chief Executive	4%	1%
Associate or Assistant	25%	28%
Administrative Assistant	19%	5%
Department Head	5%	7%
Comprehensive Health Planning	5%	5%
Governmental Health Agency	13%	35%
Long Term Care Administration	1%	2%
Mental Health Administration	2%	3%
Ambulatory Care	5%	—
Third Party Financing Agency	2%	—
Voluntary Health Agency	1%	—
Trade Association	2%	3%
University Faculty Position	4%	—
Further Graduate Study	3%	2%
Unknown/Not in Health Care	10%	8%
Total Students Reported	773	88

* Percentages rounded.

QUESTION 46 Percent faculty time devoted to continuing education

	49 U.S. Programs	5 Canadian Programs
Average	8.8%	7.0%
Range	0-51%	0-15%

QUESTION 48 Students enrolled in continuing education, number of times mentioned

	U.S.		Canadian	
	#	%*	#	%
Administrators, Health Agencies	33	28	4	31
Middle Management Personnel	28	24	4	31
Health Professionals	28	24	4	31
Consumers	13	11	1	7
Board Members	17	14	0	0
Total	119		13	

* Percentages rounded.

QUESTION 49 Financial support for continuing education, number of times mentioned

	U.S.		Canadian	
	#	%*	#	%
Federal Grants	15	21	2	22
Private Foundation Grants	14	20	1	11
University Funds	11	16	0	0
Revenue from Tuition	24	34	5	56
Other	7	10	1	11
Total	71		9	

*Percentages rounded.

QUESTION 50 Percent faculty time devoted to research

	48 U.S. Programs	4 Canadian Programs
Average	21%	18%
Range	0–60%	5–40%

QUESTION 52 Grant support for research *(last two years)**

	U.S.	Canadian
From Federal Agencies		
Number	80	8
Amount	$13,118,417	$150,000
From Private Foundations		
Number	29	1
Amount	$ 1,457,358	—

* Five programs accounted for over 50 percent of all research dollars reported.

QUESTION 54 Formal programs of service to community organizations

	49 U.S. Programs	5 Canadian Programs
Yes	65%	60%
No	35%	40%
Types of Services		
Education of consumers and other personnel from community agencies	21%	17%
Technical Assistance	32%	33%
Data Collection and Analysis	21%	17%
Management Consulting	24%	33%
Other	1%	0

QUESTION 58 Input to program objectives — Priority rankings

	U.S. Programs	Canadian Programs
Average Rank*		
Faculty	1.45	1.0
Administrators	3.32	3.4
Students	3.40	2.8
Health Professionals	3.87	4.0
Alumni	4.36	4.8
Consumers	5.47	5.4
Other	6.23	7.0

* 1 = highest rank; 7 = lowest rank

QUESTION 59 Methods of program evaluation—Times mentioned

	U.S.	Canadian
Output Evaluation		
Survey of Graduates	34	3
Survey of Employers of Graduates	20	3
Other	12	0
Input Evaluation		
Evaluation by Students	49	5
Self-assessment by Faculty	43	3
Outside Evaluation	30	1
Other	10	0

QUESTION 60 Priorities for activities other than teaching

	48 U.S. Programs	5 Canadian Programs
Average Rank*		
Research	2.8	1.8
Technical Assistance	3.0	2.2
Continuing Education (Pract. Adminis.)	3.8	3.2
Continuing Education (Alumni)	4.2	4.2
Public Policy Formulation	3.9	4.2
Special Education (Board Members)	6.1	6.4
Special Education (Consumers)	6.6	6.6
Special Education (Others)	7.4	6.6
Other	8.3	9.0

* 1 = highest rank; 9 = lowest rank.

Survey of Undergraduate Programs in Health Administration †

QUESTION 1 Type of parent institution

	Associate Degree Programs		Baccalaureate Programs		Totals	
	#	%	#	%	#	%
Public	3	60	8	62	11	61
Private	2	40	5	38	7	39

QUESTION 3 Size of parent institution measured by number of full-time undergraduate students

	Associate Degree Programs		Baccalaureate Programs		Totals	
	#	%	#	%	#	%
0–2,000 Students	4	80	—		4	22
2,001–5,000	—		6	47	6	33
5,001–10,000	—		3	23	3	17
Over 10,000	1	20	2	15	3	17
No Answer	—		2	15	2	11

QUESTION 4 Organizational locus of program within the parent college or university

	Associate Degree Programs #	Baccalaureate Programs #	Totals #
Arts and Sciences	—	1	1
Business Administration	1	3	4
Allied Health	—	3	3
Business and Public Administration	—	1	1
College of Community Services	—	1	1
College of Human Development	—	1	1
School of General Studies	—	1	1
Interdisciplinary	—	1	1
No Sub-breakdown	4	1	5

† There is not a complete sequence of questions and answers given in this paper because some were open-ended questions which did not yield quantitative answers while others did not result in significant findings.

QUESTION 6   Types of undergraduate degrees awarded by programs

	Associate Degree Programs #	Baccalaureate Programs #	Totals #
AA	3		3
AS	2	1	3
BS		11	11
BA		2	2
BBA		2	2

QUESTION 7   Overall program structure — Does your program of instruction in health administration constitute:

	Associate Degree Programs #	Baccalaureate Programs #	Totals #
A single major field of study?	4	12	16
One of multiple majors?		1	1
A minor field of study?		1	1
Others?			
Career option within AA program	1		1

QUESTION 8   Age of program — Year in which first degrees were awarded

	Associate Degree Programs #	Baccalaureate Programs #	Totals #
None yet awarded	1	4	5
1973		2	2
1972	1	2	3
1971		2	2
1970		1	1
1969			
1968	1		1
1967	1	1	2
1966		1	1

QUESTION 11 University owned or operated health facilities (excluding student infirmaries)

	Associate Degree Programs #	Baccalaureate Programs #	Totals #
Do you have such facilities?			
Yes	0	5	5
No	5	8	13
If yes, are they used in your teaching program?			
Yes		5	5
No		0	0

QUESTION 12 Number of students enrolled in the programs

	Associate Degree Programs #	Associate Degree Programs %	Baccalaureate Programs #	Baccalaureate Programs %	Totals #	Totals %
a. Full-time Students						
Total	44		477		521	
Mean	9		10		31	
Range	0–17		1–128		0–128	
b. Part-time Students						
Total	42		14		56	
Mean	8		1		3	
Range	0–20		0–5		0–20	
c. Breakdown by Sex						
Total Male Students	44	57	339	69	383	67
Total Female Students	33	43	152	31	185	33
d. Minority Group Students						
Black	2	2	60	12	62	11
Spanish Surname	4	5	10	3	14	2
Native American	0	00	2	<1	2	
e. Continuing Education Students not enrolled for credit	77		43		120	
f. Non-degree Students taking some courses for credit	22		46		68	

QUESTION 13 Age distribution of students

	Associate Degree Programs		Baccalaureate Programs		Totals	
	#	%	#	%	#	%
Under 25	17	40	395	73	412	70
25–35	17	40	120	22	137	24
Over 35	9	20	28	5	37	6

QUESTION 16 Students' work experience prior to entering programs*

	Associate Degree Programs #	Baccalaureate Programs #	Totals #	%
Full-Time Students				
a. Health Administration	6	52	58	25
b. Nursing Practice	3	17	20	9
c. Other—Health related	2	101	103	45
d. Other—Non-health related	9	38	47	21
Part-Time Students				
a. Health Administration	15	—	15	29
b. Nursing Practice	4	6	10	20
c. Other—Health related	4	10	14	27
d. Other—Non-health related	8	4	12	24

* There were a substantial number of "no responses" to this question.

QUESTION 19 Percentage of program students who complete programs of study and receive their degrees

	Associate Degree Programs %	Baccalaureate Programs %	Totals %
Average Percentage	77	85	82
Range of Percentages	60–90	30–100	30–100
	N=3	N=7	N=10

QUESTION 21a Number of full-time program faculty members by sex and academic rank

	Associate Degree Programs #	Baccalaureate Programs #	Totals #
Full Professor			
Male	0	3	3
Female	0	1	1
Associate Professor, Tenured			
Male	1	0	1
Female	0	0	0
Associate Professor, Non-tenured			
Male	0	4	4
Female	1	1	2
Assistant Professor			
Male	2	14	16
Female	0	1	1
Other (Instructor, Lecturer, etc.)			
Male	3	8	11
Female	1	2	3
	N=5	N=12	
Average Number of Full-time Faculty Members per Program	1.6	2.8	2.5

QUESTION 21b Number of part-time program faculty members

	Associate Degree Programs #	Baccalaureate Programs #	Totals #	%
Male Part-time Faculty	12	34	46	84
Female Part-time Faculty	3	6	9	16
Total	15	40	55	
	N=5	N=12	N=17	
Average number of part-time faculty members per program	3.0	3.3	3.2	

QUESTION 22 Program director: rank and highest degree

	Associate Degree Programs #	Baccalaureate Programs #	Totals #	%
a. Rank				
Professor	0	3	3	18
Associate Professor	2	1	3	18
Assistant Professor	1	6	7	41
Other	2	2	4	23
b. Highest Degree Held				
PhD	0	2	2	
MD	0	0	0	
Other doctors'	1	3	4	
MPH	0	0	0	
MHA	1	3	4	
Other master's	2	3	5	
Bachelor's	1	1	2	

QUESTION 24 Full-time program faculty: degrees held and areas of specialization*

	Associate Degree Programs #	Baccalaureate Programs #	Totals #	%
Doctoral Degree Holders				
Health/Hospital Administration	0	6	6	
Medical Care Organization	0	3	3	
Economics	1	2	3	
Management/Organization Theory	0	2	2	
Other	0	2	2	
Total			16	33
Master's/Bachelor's Degree Holders				
Health/Hospital Administration	1	8	9	
Medical Care Organization	0	1	1	
Economics/Financial Mgmt.	2	1	3	
Management/Organization Theory	3	3	6	
Comprehensive Health Planning	0	4	4	
Other	0	9	9	
Total			32	67

* Figures as reported for this question do not reconcile in total with those of Question 21a due to the discrepancies in the data reported on the questionnaires.

QUESTION 25 Program budgets*

	Associate Degree Programs N=3	Baccalaureate Programs N=11	Totals N=14
Total Budget From All Sources			
Total	$62,000	$2,167,000	$2,229,000
Average	21,000	197,000	159,000
Range	5–32,000	23–429,000	5–429,000
Breakdown—Average Amounts budgeted for			
Teaching	12,000	110,000	89,000
Student Support	300	33,000	26,000
Research	700	15,000	12,000
Continuing Education	5,000	10,000	9,000
Other	3,000	29,000	23,000

* Includes Navy—G.W. Program not included in main report.

QUESTION 26 Source of funds

	Associate Degree Programs		Baccalaureate Programs	
	#	%	#	%
Federal Grants	—		$ 964,000	45
State Government	—		518,000	24
Private Foundations	—		45,000	2
Internal University Funds	$62,000	100	180,000	8
Other	—		460,000	21
Total	$62,000	100	$2,167,000	100
	N=3		N=11	

QUESTION 28 Typical program curriculum structure: average number of credit hours for each category shown*

	Associate Degree Programs		Baccalaureate Programs	
	#	%	#	%
a. Required courses in health administration	16	21	22	17
b. Elective courses in health administration	1	1	9	7
c. Required courses in fields directly related to health administration	18	24	28	22
d. Elective courses in fields directly related to health administration	6	8	10	8
e. Required courses other than a and c above (e.g. general education courses)	23	31	41	31
f. Elective courses other than b and d above	11	15	20	15
Total	75	100	130	100

* Units are credit hours.

QUESTION 29 Specialty tracks in the program curriculum

	Associate Degree Programs #	Baccalaureate Programs #	Totals #
a. Functional Specialty Tracks			
Financial Management	1	3	4
Planning	1	4	5
Personnel Administration	1	3	4
Systems Analysis	0	2	2
Policy Analysis	0	1	1
Communications	1	1	2
b. Organizational or Program Specialty Tracks			
Ambulatory Care Admin.	0	4	4
Hospital Administration	0	5	5
Long Term Care Admin.	2	5	7
Mental Health Admin.	0	2	2
Public Health Admin.	0	3	3

QUESTION 30 Curriculum content areas: required courses in health administration*

	Associate Degree Programs #	Baccalaureate Programs #	Totals #
General—Health Admin.	8	14	22
Hospital Administration	8	7	15
Medical Care Organization	2	9	11
Public Health—Epidemiology	0	7	7
Financial Management	1	5	6
Systems/Quantitative Methods	0	6	6
Health Planning	0	4	4
Health Economics	0	4	4
Personnel Administration/ Labor Relations	1	2	3
Law	2	1	3
Long Term Care Admin.	1	1	2
Medical Sociology	0	2	2
Purchasing/Materials/ Plant Management	0	2	2

* Units: Number of required courses.

QUESTION 31 Curriculum content areas: elective courses in health administration

	Associate Degree Programs #	Baccalaureate Programs #	Totals #
Medical Care Organization	2	3	5
Systems/Quantitative Methods	0	4	4
General—Health Admin.	0	3	3
Planning	0	3	3
Long Term Care Admin.	0	3	3
Law	0	3	3
Medical Sociology	0	2	2
Hospital Administration	0	1	1
Personnel Administration	0	2	2
Financial Management	0	1	1
Materials Management	0	1	1

QUESTION 32 Field experience components of the curriculum

	Associate Degree Programs #	Baccalaureate Programs #	Totals #
Administrative residency			
0–3 months	2	6	8
4–6	0	2	2
Continuous part-time field experience concurrent with on-campus study	3	3	6

QUESTION 37 Total number of program graduates to date

	Associate Degree Programs #	Baccalaureate Programs #	Totals #
Total	32	405	437
Average Number per Program	16	45	40
	N=2	N=9	N=11
No Graduates as Yet	2	3	5
No Answer to Question	1	1	2

QUESTION 39 Undergraduate placement data

	Associate Degree Programs %	Baccalaureate Programs %
Hospital Administration	22%	51%
Chief Executive	—	5%
Associate or Assistant	—	5%
Administrative Assistant	—	27%
Department Head	—	14%
Comprehensive Health Planning	—	10%
Government Health Agency	—	5%
Long Term Care Admin.	78%	5%
Ambulatory Care	—	4%
Third-Party Financing	—	—
Voluntary Health Agency	—	3%
Trade Association	—	—
Further Study	—	22%
Total Students Reported	N=9	N=135

QUESTION 41 Continuing education activities of the undergraduate programs

	Associate Degree Programs #	Baccalaureate Programs #	Totals #	%
Is your program involved in continuing education?				
Yes	3	8	11	61
No	2	5	7	39
Total number of continuing education courses offered during last two years	7	17	24	
Kinds of students who enrolled (number of times mentioned)				
Administrators	3	4	7	
Health professionals	2	4	6	
Board members		1	1	
Consumers		1	1	

QUESTION 42 Research activities

	Associate Degree Programs #	Baccalaureate Programs #	Totals #	%
Is your faculty engaged in research activities?				
Yes	1	7	8	44
No	4	6	10	56
Number and total amount of research grants received within the last two years		4–$171,000		

QUESTION 43 Community service activities

	Associate Degree Programs #	Baccalaureate Programs #	Totals #	%
Is your program involved in any formally constituted programs of service to community organizations?				
Yes	0	8	8	44
No	5	5	10	56
Types of service provided				
Education of consumers and other personnel from community agencies		3		
Technical assistance		7		
Data collection and analysis		3		
Management consulting		3		
Other		1		

QUESTION 48 Reasons for starting an undergraduate program in health administration

	Associate Degree Programs #	Baccalaureate Programs #	Totals #	%
a. To attract more students to parent college or university				
Very important	0	1	1	6
Important	2	2	4	22
Minor consideration	3	10	13	72
b. To fill manpower shortages in your community or region				
Very important	5	9	14	78
Important	1	3	4	22
Minor consideration	0	0	0	0
c. To develop a "new breed" of administrators				
Very important	2	6	8	47
Important	2	3	5	29
Minor consideration	1	3	4	24
d. To provide entry opportunities for minority group members				
Very important	0	3	3	17
Important	2	4	6	33
Minor consideration	3	6	9	50

QUESTION 50 Input into formulation of program's educational objectives and policies — Priority rankings*

	Associate Degree Programs	Baccalaureate Programs	Totals
Average Ranking			
Practicing administrators in the community	1.4	3.0	2.6
Faculty	4.2	2.2	2.7
Health professionals in the community	2.4	3.7	3.3
Students	4.8	3.5	3.8
Consumers of health services	4.8	5.2	5.1
Others	5.8	5.5	5.6
Alumni of the program	6.4	6.0	6.1

* 1=Greatest Input   7=Least Input

QUESTION 52 Priority rankings for activities other than undergraduate teaching*

	Associate Degree Programs	Baccalaureate Programs	Totals
Average Ranking			
Continuing education for practicing administrators in the community	1.4	3.0	2.5
Continuing education for program graduates	1.6	3.7	3.1
Technical assistance to community agencies	4.0	3.6	3.7
Public policy formulation	4.8	5.2	5.1
Research in health services delivery and administration	6.4	4.6	5.1
Special education for others	7.6	5.3	6.0
Special education for board members	6.6	6.1	6.3
Special education for consumers	5.6	6.8	6.4
Other	8.4	8.8	8.6

*1=Highest priority   9=Lowest priority

Survey of Students in Graduate Programs †
(Academic Year 1972-73)

QUESTION 1 Distribution by sex

	Number	Percentage
Male	697	84.7
Female	126	15.3

QUESTION 2 Age of students

Age in Years	Percentage Frequency
<26	14.7
26-30	45.7
31-40	30.7
41-50	6.8
51-60	1.2

QUESTION 3 Ethnic background

	Percentage Frequency
Black	4.1
Mexican American	.2
Caucasian	90.0
Oriental	.7
American Indian	.7
Puerto Rican	1.0
Other	3.2

QUESTION 4 Educational background

(a) Highest degree obtained prior to graduate program

	Percentage Frequency
PhD	.2
Master's	16.7
MD	2.9
Bachelor's	78.0
Other Doctorate	2.2

(b) Undergraduate major

	Percentage Frequency
Health related	28.1
Non-health related (business or management)	32.4
Non-health related (not business or management)	39.5

† There is not a complete sequence of questions and answers given in this paper because some were open-ended questions which did not yield quantitative answers while others did not result in significant findings.

QUESTION 5 Occupational history

(a) Prior to entering graduate program, did you have any full-time work experience?

Work Experience	Yes	Mean No. of Years
Health related	61.4%	5.48
Non-health related	60.5%	4.11

(b) Highest annual salary prior to graduate program

	Percentage Frequency
Less than $5,000	18.9
$ 5,000– 9,999	32.4
$10,000–14,999	32.9
$15,000–19,999	12.4
$20,000–24,999	2.2
$25,000 or more	1.2

QUESTION 6 Educational expenses*

Percentage of Students Who Spent Line Amount in Various Categories

Amount Spent in Various Categories	Tuition and fees	Books and supplies	Room and board	Personal and other expenses
Less than $1,000	13.4	96.3	11.0	29.4
$1,000–1,999	21.7	3.4	15.5	28.4
$2,000–2,999	26.4	0.2	23.3	18.2
$3,000–3,999	20.1	0.2	17.8	8.1
$4,000–4,999	18.3	0.0	32.4	16.0

* Percentages rounded.

QUESTION 6(b) Sources of support while enrolled in graduate program

	Percentage Frequency
Family, Relatives	7.43
Self, Spouse	35.52
Employer	12.21
University Scholarship or Fellowship	3.75
Loans	5.40
Veterans Benefits (GI bills)	6.86
Residency stipend	10.19
Grants	
a. PHS traineeship	10.19
b. Other grant funds	2.48
Other Sources	3.38

QUESTION 7 Degree of emphasis and relevance for each subject in your program

(a) Mean Scores

1 = High
2 = Moderate
3 = Low
4 = None

	Emphasis	Relevance
General administration and organization theory	1.75	1.55
Administrative and organization theory applied to health services organizations	1.78	1.41
Medical care organization	1.87	1.58
Principles of medical and nursing practice	3.01	2.24
Public health practice and community medicine	2.53	2.07
Comprehensive health planning	2.05	1.74
Financial management	2.32	1.29
Personnel administration	2.83	1.82
Computer application—systems analysis	2.64	1.97
Quantitative methods—applied statistics	2.00	1.97
Economic theory	2.48	2.13
Industrial relations	3.13	2.28
Research methodology	2.33	2.26
Health law	2.52	1.67
Medical sociology	2.76	2.26
Epidemiology	2.75	2.52
Political science–government relations	2.96	2.01

(b) Strongest and weakest areas in curriculum

Three Strongest Areas

(1) Administrative and organizational theory applied to health services organizations
(2) General administrative and organizational theory
(3) Medical care organization

Three Weakest Areas

(1) Financial management
(2) Health law
(3) Computer applications-systems analysis

QUESTION 8 Did program offer opportunity to select course work?

	Percentage Frequency
High flexibility	22.41
Moderate	41.13
Very little	31.90
None	4.56

QUESTION 9 Did graduate program include a formal residency or field experience component?

	Percentage
Yes	89.0
No	11.0

(b) How long was residency in months?

Mean	8.48 months
Range	1 to 32 months
Mode	12 months

(c) This residency period of time was

	Percentage Frequency
Too long	9.7
Too short	15.9
About right	74.4

(d) Overall evaluation of field experience

	Percentage Frequency
Very valuable—the most important part of your program	44.2
Valuable—of equal importance to academic work	43.2
Of some value but less than academic work	9.6
Of minimum value	2.9

QUESTION 10 Would residency have better qualified you for entry into health administration field if you had had one?

	Percentage Frequency
Strongly agree	38.3
Agree	23.4
Disagree	17.8
Strongly disagree	12.1
No opinion	8.4

QUESTION 11 Did your program require completion of specific educational prerequisites prior to admission?

	Percentage
Yes	63.3
No	36.7

(b) With regard to educational prerequisites

	Percentage Frequency
Minimal requirements to encourage diversity in student backgrounds	55.0
Upgraded—require greater number of successfully mastered prerequisites	24.1
Standardized—specific undergraduate degrees or background requirement	8.3
Both standardized and upgraded	12.7

QUESTION 12 Program organization, facilities, and resources

Mean Scores
- 1 = Needs improvement
- 2 = Satisfactory
- 3 = Above average
- 4 = Superior

	Adequency	Effective use by faculty and students
Library facilities	2.54	2.54
Computer facilities	2.44	2.01
Community resources	2.98	2.45
Curriculum integration	1.92	
Relevance of curriculum to health care stystem	2.24	
Number of full-time faculty	2.00	
Supplementary education programs	2.61	
Faculty-Student interaction	2.13	
Financial assistance programs for students	1.92	
Program support to graduates	1.90	

QUESTION 13 Degree of difficulty in finding a job

	Percentage Frequency
No difficulty	40.6
Little difficulty	16.9
Moderate difficulty	24.8
Considerable difficulty	17.8

QUESTION 14 Overall quality of graduate education

	Percentage Frequency
Needs improvement	19.9
Satisfactory	26.2
Above average	38.4
Superior	15.6

QUESTION 15 Administrative specialization with an area of subject specialization

	Percentage Frequency
Strongly agree	25.3
Agree	42.1
Disagree	23.8
Strongly disagree	8.7

(b) If you strongly agree or agree to subject specialization, which specialty areas should be offered?

	Percentage Frequency
Financial management	59.1
Planning	49.2
Systems analysis	40.8
Personnel administration	31.3
Policy analysis	23.7
Communications	16.6

(c) Do you see need for programs of institutional specialization within graduate programs?

	Percentage Frequency
Strongly agree	17.1
Agree	38.0
Disagree	33.7
Strongly disagree	11.2

QUESTION 16 Given limited resources, assign priorities for particular programs *(1=highest, 9=lowest)*

(1) Continuing education of program graduates
(2) Continuing education of practicing administrators who are not program graduates
(3) Research in health services delivery and administration
(4) Technical assistance and consultation to community health agencies
(5) Involvement in public policy formation
(6) Special educational opportunities for board members
(7) Special educational opportunities for consumers
(8) Special educational opportunities for others
(9) Other

QUESTION 17 Sources of input for educational program planning and design *(1=highest, 7=lowest)*

(1) Practicing administrators in the community
(2) Faculty
(3) Alumni
(4) Health professionals
(5) Students
(6) Consumers
(7) Others

QUESTION 18 Reaction to following statements

Mean Scores
- 1 = Strongly agree
- 2 = Agree
- 3 = Disagree
- 4 = Strongly disagree

	Agreement	Disagreement
Graduate programs should primarily be concerned with entry-level positions		2.87
Development of undergraduate programs should be encouraged for middle-management positions	2.20	
Health administration should be licensed by governmental agency		2.85
Professional association should require mandatory continuing education professional exams	2.03	
University programs should attempt to influence values of students		2.56
Minimum standards of quality need be established and programs evaluated by outside agency	1.74	

Survey of 1971 Alumni of Graduate Programs †

QUESTION 1   Distribution by sex

	Number	Percentage
Male	369	84.8
Female	66	15.2

QUESTION 2   Age

Age in Years	Percentage Frequency
<26	.5
26–30	32.3
31–40	49.7
41–50	14.4
51–60	3.0
–61	.2

QUESTION 3   Ethnic Background

	Percentage Frequency
Black	2.8
Mexican American	.2
Caucasian	91.8
Oriental	1.6
American Indian	.5
Puerto Rican	1.6
Other	1.4

QUESTION 4   Educational background

(a) Highest degree obtained prior to graduate program

	Percentage Frequency
PhD	.5
Master's	19.1
MD	4.9
Bachelor's	73.5
Other	2.1

(b) Undergraduate major

	Percentage Frequency
Health related	35%
Non-health related in business or management	30%
Non-health related not in business or management	35%

† There is not a complete sequence of questions and answers given in this paper because some were open-ended questions which did not yield quantitative answers while others did not result in significant findings.

QUESTION 5 Occupational history

(a) Prior to entering graduate program did you have any full-time work experience?

Work Experience	Yes	Mean No. of Years
Health related	70.3%	6.36
Non-health related	63.1%	4.14

(b) Highest annual salary achieved prior to entry into graduate program

	Percentage Frequency
Less than $5,000	16.1
$ 5,000– 9,999	39.0
$10,000–14,999	31.2
$15,000–19,999	7.6
$20,000–24,999	3.2
$25,000 or more	2.9

QUESTION 6 Estimated direct cost of graduate studies

Amount Spent in Various Categories	Percentage of Students Who Spent Line Amount in Various Categories			
	Tuition and fees	Books and supplies	Room and board	Personal and other expenses
Less than $1,000	18.6	93.0	11.0	26.3
$1,000–1,999	26.7	6.5	15.1	27.9
$2,000–2,999	28.8	.2	20.4	18.3
$3,000–3,999	13.7	0.0	18.7	9.9
4,000 or more	12.1	0.0	34.8	17.6

(b) Sources of support while enrolled in graduate program

	Percentage Frequency
Family, relatives	7.22
Self, spouse	35.36
Employer	13.27
University scholarship or fellowship	2.80
Loans	3.98
Veterans benefits (GI bills)	5.38
Residency stipend	6.81
Grants	
a. PHS traineeship	15.21
b. Other grant funds	2.37
Other sources	3.75

QUESTION 7 Degree of emphasis and relevance for each subject area in your program

Mean scores
1 = High
2 = Moderate
3 = Low
4 = None

	Emphasis	Relevance
General administrative and organizational theory	1.74	1.57
Administrative and organizational theory applied to health services organizations	1.71	1.57
Medical care organization	1.80	1.70
Principles of medical and nursing practice	2.97	2.25
Comprehensive health planning	2.14	2.15
Financial management	2.48	1.70
Personnel administration	2.72	1.89
Computer applications–systems analysis	2.72	2.28
Quantitative methods–applied statistics	2.20	2.34
Economic theory	2.52	2.57
Industrial relations	3.04	2.57
Research methodology	2.32	2.43
Health law	2.44	2.07
Medical sociology	2.64	2.43
Epidemiology	2.73	2.86
Political science–government relations	2.98	2.24
Public health and community medicine	2.44	2.38

(b) Strongest and weakest areas in curriculum

Three Strongest Areas
   (1) Administrative and organizational theory applied to health services organizations
   (2) General administrative and organizational theory
   (3) Medical care organization

Three Weakest Areas
   (1) Financial management
   (2) Computer applications-systems analysis
   (3) Personnel administration

QUESTION 8 Did program offer opportunity to select course work?

	Percentage Frequency
High flexibility	23.5
Moderate flexibility	36.6
Very little flexibility	30.4
None	9.4

QUESTION 9 Did graduate program have a formal residency or field experience component?

(a) Did graduate program have a formal residency?

	Percentage
Yes	91.0
No	9.0

(b) How long was residency in months?

Mean	8.66 months
Median	9.36 months

Ninety-eight percent of those having a formal residency indicated that the residency was longer than one month but less than one year.

(c) This residency period of time was

	Percentage Frequency
Too long	8.7
Too short	12.8
About right	78.5

(d) Overall evaluation of field experience

	Percentage Frequency
Very valuable—the most important part of your program	32.0
Valuable—of equal importance to academic work	44.8
Of some value but less than academic work	17.9
Of minimum value	5.4

QUESTION 10 Of the nine percent respondents who had no formal residency program, 40.4 percent agreed and 36.2 percent disagreed that a field experience component would have better qualified them for entry into their present position

	Percentage Frequency
Strongly agree	17.0
Agree	23.4
Disagree	36.2
Strongly disagree	21.3
No opinion	2.1

QUESTION 11 Did your program require completion of specific educational prerequisites prior to admission?

	Percentage Frequency
Yes	67.3
No	32.7

(b) With regard to educational prerequisites

	Percentage Frequency
Minimal requirements—to encourage diversity in student backgrounds	55.7
Upgraded—require greater number of successfully mastered prerequisites	19.6
Standardized—specific undergraduate degrees or background required	9.7
Both standardized and upgraded	15.0

QUESTION 12 Program organization, facilities, and resources

Mean Scores
- 1 = Needs improvement
- 2 = Satisfactory
- 3 = Above average
- 4 = Superior

	Availability	Effective use by students and faculty
Library facilities	2.87	2.77
Computer facilties	2.25	1.88
Community resources	2.98	2.27
Curriculum integration	2.08	
Relevancy of curriculum to health care system	2.34	
Number of full-time faculty	2.16	
Faculty-student interaction	2.31	
Supplementary educational programs	2.69	
Financial assistance programs for students	2.21	
Program support to graduates	1.97	

QUESTION 13 Search for employment

(c) Did job meet your original expectations?

	Percentage
Yes	63.9
Only partly	25.2
No	10.9

(d) Degree of difficulty in finding job

	Percentage
None	47.4
Little	20.9
Moderate	21.4
Considerable	10.3

QUESTION 14 Overall quality of graduate education

	Percentage Frequency
Needs improvement	17.7
Satisfactory	23.2
Above average	42.8
Superior	16.3

QUESTION 15 Administrative specialization with an area of subject specialization

Strongly agree	21.2
Agree	41.2
Disagree	25.8
Strongly disagree	11.9

(b) If you strongly agree or agree to subject specialization, which specialty areas should be offered?

	Percentage Frequency
Financial management	52.2
Planning	41.8
Personnel administration	28.0
Communications	17.5
Systems analysis	34.7
Policy analysis	20.9

(c) Do you see need for programs of institutional specialization within graduate programs?

	Percentage Frequency
Strongly agree	13.5
Agree	38.1
Disagree	35.0
Strongly disagree	13.5

QUESTION 16 Given limited resources, assign priorities for particular programs *(1=highest, 9=lowest)*

(1) Continuing education of program graduates
(2) Continuing education of practicing administrators who are not program graduates
(3) Research in health services delivery and administration
(4) Technical assistance and consultation to community health agencies
(5) Involvement in public policy formation
(6) Special educational opportunities for board members
(7) Special educational opportunities for consumers
(8) Special educational opportunities for others
(9) Other

QUESTION 17 Sources of input for educational program planning and design *(1=highest, 7=lowest)*

(1) Practicing administrators in the community
(2) Faculty
(3) Alumni
(4) Health professionals
(5) Students
(6) Consumers
(7) Other

QUESTION 18 Reactions to following statements

Mean Scores
   (1) Strongly agree
   (2) Agree
   (3) Disagree
   (4) Strongly disagree

	Agree	Disagree
Graduate programs should primarily be concerned with entry-level positions		2.93
Development of undergraduate programs should be encouraged for middle-management positions	2.17	
Health administrators should be licensed by governmental agency		2.96
Professional associations should require mandatory continuing education +/− professional exams	2.01	
University programs should attempt to influence values of students	2.40	
Minimum standards of quality need to be established and programs evaluated by outside agency	1.76	

QUESTION 19 Describe organization

	Percentage Frequency
Acute hospital facility	49.0
Long term care facility	2.3
Mental health facility	2.8
Medical clinic	3.7
CHP agency	4.6
State or local PH dept.	3.7
Health insurance organization	1.1
Regional medical program	1.4
Medical foundation	0.2
Other	29.0

QUESTION 19(b) Approximate population of the community in which your institution is located

	Percentage Frequency
Less than 8,000	3.1
8,000– 59,999	13.4
60,000–149,999	17.2
150,000–999,999	36.3
1,000,000 or more	30.0

Survey of Employers of the 1971 Alumni †

QUESTION 3 Date of birth

Age in Years	Percentage Frequency
<26	0.4
26–30	2.1
31–40	29.0
41–50	41.1
51–60	17.4
–61	6.2

QUESTION 4 Distribution by sex

	Number	Percentage
Male	215	90.3
Female	23	9.7

QUESTION 5 Educational background

(a) Highest degree obtained

	Percentage Frequency
PhD	5.1
Master's	66.8
MD	14.5
Bachelor's	9.8
Other	3.8

(b) Undergraduate Major

	Percentage Frequency
Health related	39
Non-health related (business or management)	29
Non-health related (not business or management)	32

(c) If you hold a master's degree, your major field

	Percentage Frequency
Hospital administration	56.8
Public health administration	11.4
Medical care organization	4.3
Health planning	2.2
Business administration	4.9
Other	20.0

† There is not a complete sequence of questions and answers given in this paper because some were open-ended questions which did not yield quantitative answers while others did not result in significant findings.

QUESTION 6 In addition to person giving you this questionnaire, have you worked with other graduates of health administration or planning programs?

	Percentage
Yes	93.4
No	6.2

QUESTIONS 7 and 9 Types of positions held by graduates and vacancies graduates would be hired to fill*

	Type of positions held by graduates	Types of vacancies graduates hired to fill
Top-level management	68.9%	78.4%
Middle-level management	50.2%	74.3%
Supervisory-first level	14.1%	26.1%
Staff assistant or analyst	29.9%	48.1%

* Percentages in the first column are of respondents having graduates holding the indicated levels of positions; the second column (right) shows percentages of respondents who would hire graduates to fill vacancies at the indicated levels.

QUESTION 8 When vacancies for administrative personnel exist in your organization do you prefer to hire graduates of health administration (or planning) programs to fill these positions?

	Percentage
Yes	92.4
No	7.6

QUESTION 10 Knowledge and skill area

Mean Scores

1 = High
2 = Moderate
3 = Low
4 = None

	Degree required by graduate	Degree the graduate is qualified
Administrative and organization theory	1.34	1.41
Medical care organization	1.30	1.40
Quantitative methods/applied statistics	1.85	1.87
Public health administration	2.20	1.92
Comprehensive health planning	1.77	1.67
Personnel administration	1.37	1.76
Systems analysis/computer applications	2.33	2.31
Financial management	1.60	1.96
Research methodology	1.55	1.65
Law	1.95	2.00
Industrial relations	2.35	2.28
Epidemiology	2.70	2.32
Medical sociology	2.04	1.87
Political science/government relations	1.75	1.81
Medical/nursing practice	1.67	1.62

QUESTION 11 Most crucial and most deficient knowledge and skill areas in order of importance

Most crucial

(1) Administrative and organization theory
(2) Medical care organization
(3) Financial management
(4) Personnel administration

Most deficient

(1) Financial management
(2) Personnel administration
(3) Research methodology
(4) Industrial relations

QUESTION 12 How well prepared was this graduate?

Ninety-four percent felt the graduate was highly (1) or moderately well (2) prepared with the mean of the distribution falling at 1.6 and standard deviation of .6

(a) Do you have other administrative personnel in your organization at approximately the same level of responsibility as the program graduate, who have not had formal education in health administration or planning?

	Percentage
Yes	63
No	37

(b) If yes, was the graduate better prepared than individual with no formal training?

	Percentage Frequency
Strongly agree	34.9
Agree	45.4
Disagree	17.1
Strongly disagree	2.6

QUESTION 13 Graduate program concerned primarily with entry level positions

	Percentage Frequency
Strongly agree	21.8
Agree	50.4
Disagree	22.6
Strongly disagree	5.1

(b) Emphasis on "Future Executive Approach"

	Percentage Frequency
Strongly agree	27.8
Agree	51.5
Disagree	19.0
Strongly disagree	1.7

QUESTION 14 Favor subject specialization

	Percentage Frequency
Strongly agree	17.9
Agree	48.7
Disagree	30.8
Strongly disagree	2.6

(b) Of the 67 percent who agreed or strongly agreed to having Subject Specialization, the following percentages indicate the speciality areas which should be offered

Speciality Area	Percentage Frequency
Financial management	54.8
Planning	47.7
Personnel administration	41.5
Communications	22.4
Systems analysis	39.4
Policy analysis	25.3

(c) Need for institutional specialization

	Percentage Frequency
Strongly agree	10.3
Agree	35.0
Disagree	46.2
Strongly disagree	8.5

QUESTION 15 On-the-job training essential prior to graduate entering field

	Percentage Frequency
Strongly agree	58.7
Agree	29.4
Disagree	11.5
Strongly disagree	0.4

QUESTION 16 Of the 88 percent who agreed or strongly agreed that a period of on-the-job training was essential, they were about evenly divided as to who should assume the responsibility with 45.2 percent assigning it to the profession of practicing administrators and 54.8 percent relegating this responsibility to the universities.

QUESTION 17 Types of residencies or field experience beneficial

	Percentage Frequency
Rotation—whereby a student rotates through the various departments etc., of an organization for orientation purposes	52.7
Project oriented—whereby the student is assigned an array of specific projects to complete	52.3
Specific assignment—whereby the student is given a specific job or function(s) for the course of his residency or field experience	30.3
Intermittent—whereby the student would spend varying amounts of time per week in an organization during the period he or she is completing the academic portion of the program (i.e. part-time residency integrated with academic work).	36.1
Multiple institution—whereby the student rotates among a number of different kinds of health care organizations	38.2

QUESTION 18 Given limited resources, priorities for programs were assigned in this order

(1) Continuing education of program graduates
(2) Continuing education of practicing administrators who were not program graduates
(3) Research in health services delivery and administration
(4) Technical assistance and consultation to community health agencies
(5) Special education opportunities for board members
(6) Involvement in public policy formation
(7) Special educational opportunities for consumers
(8) Special educational opportunities for others
(9) Other

QUESTION 19 Sources of input for educational program planning and design

(1) Practicing administrators in the community
(2) Faculty
(3) Health professionals
(4) Alumni
(5) Students
(6) Consumers
(7) Other

QUESTION 20 Reactions to statements

(a) Health administrators should be licensed by a governmental agency

	Percentage Frequency
Strongly agree	10.2
Agree	24.7
Strongly disagree	34.5
Disagree	30.6

(b) Continuing education and/or professional exams for membership criteria for professional association

	Percentage Frequency
Strongly agree	36.0
Agree	44.1
Strongly disagree	13.6
Disagree	6.4

(c) University programs should attempt to influence values of students

	Percentage Frequency
Strongly agree	22.4
Agree	51.3
Strongly disagree	19.7
Disagree	6.6

(d) Minimum standards of quality should be established and programs should be evaluated by outside agency

	Percentage Frequency
Strongly agree	38.3
Agree	49.4
Strongly disagree	7.7
Disagree	4.7

Part III

Report of a
Field Research Study

Authors in Part III

Robert F. Allison, Ph.D.
Assistant Professor of Hospital Administration
School of Public Health
University of Michigan

William L. Dowling, Ph.D.
Associate Professor and Director
  Graduate Program in Health Services
  Administration and Planning
School of Public Health and Community Medicine
University of Washington

Fred C. Munson, Ph.D.
Professor of Hospital Administration
  and Research Associate in Population Planning
School of Public Health
University of Michigan

The Role of the Health Services Administrator and Implications for Educators*

The size and growth of an industry currently comprising eight percent of the nation's Gross National Product has generated an interest in effective and efficient delivery of health services. Those who provide much of the money to pay for health services are understandably interested in the stewardship of such funds exercised by executives of health service delivery organizations. Patients, consumer groups, and the general public are equally interested in the social responsibility of leaders in an industry characterized by problems concerning distribution and access of health care. Managers of these delivery organizations who find themselves between the conflicting demands of third parties desiring efficiency and patients desiring effectiveness are likewise interested in how successful executives manage such diverse and conflicting demands. Educators devoted to the preparation of such executives are concerned with understanding the real and ideal roles of management in delivery organizations as well as the educational preparation recommended for such roles. The research conducted in 1973 and reported here was an attempt to provide some answers for these diverse groups interested in the leadership role in delivery organizations and to extend certain theories of organization to a role study.

Twenty-four chief executive officers completed questionnaires and were given structured interviews. There were six respondents in each of four types of delivery organizations i.e., hospitals, long-term care facilities (LTC), multi-specialty group practice clinics, and health maintenance organizations of the prepaid group practice type (HMO's).

Since we were interested in the role of "successful" chief executives,

---

* by Robert F. Allison, William L. Dowling, and Fred C. Munson. The work leading to the report was supported by U.S. Department of H.E.W. contract HSM 110-73-437.

both the research sites and respondents were selected on the basis of meeting certain criteria of success. Principal criteria for organizational excellence included accreditation and licensure where applicable, and reputation among knowledgeable sources within the relevant industry. Criteria for successful executives included membership and offices held within the relevant professional society and reputation among leaders within the relevant industry. The assumption was made that successful executives would be associated with organizations of recognized quality.

Specifically, our study sought to achieve the following objectives: develop a methodology for describing and analyzing executives roles; develop a more detailed understanding of the administrative role in organizations; identify the key determinants of the roles studied; and identify the sources of obtaining the competence required to perform the roles.

A problem in empirical research is the time-bound nature of the data. That is, considering the rate of change, of what relevance to education of future executives is information about today's executives? One approach is to make prognostications about the future and deduce the future role from such assumptions. Another, nonempirical approach is to conceptualize the ideal role devoid of assumptions about the situational context. In our research, we took a middle course in solving this problem. We identified the leading edge of growth in the field today and chose our organizations accordingly. Because the average size of hospitals is growing, we selected one-half of the hospitals from the over 400 bed size category. The rapid growth in group practice medical clinics led to the inclusion of this type organization. Since HMO's are currently in favor and growing in size and numbers, they too were included. Traditionally, long-term care facilities have been of the owner-operator, "ma and pa" type. Recent growth of corporate chains in this industry led us to choose one-half of our sample of LTC facilities from each of these two subtypes. The relevance of our data depends on the assumptions one makes of the future. If one assumes HMO's are the organizational form of the future, our data on present HMO's may be of value in conceptualizing the future role within that type organization.

A second approach we took to the time limitations of a role study was to address the question of role determinants i.e., cause and effect. If one knows the present causal factors influencing roles, by making assumptions about the future value of causal determinants, predictions of future effects (i.e., roles) is possible. It was necessary, therefore, to specify a theory of role determination. We address now the theoretical perspective guiding this comparative study of executives roles.

Theoretical Perspective

There has been no lack of research into the nature of executive roles in delivery organizations, but much of it has suffered from one or more deficiencies. Perhaps the most basic deficiency has been what Bennis described as viewing "organizations without people" or "people without organizations."[1] Studies which have proceeded from a theoretical perspective have commonly used a closed-system or mechanistic view of organizational reality. Such studies assume given organizational goals and view the executive function as determining organizational structure and carrying out "management functions" such as planning, organizing, staffing, directing, and control.[2]

More practical problems arise from the difficulty in interpretation and utilization of the units of analysis recommended by such perspectives. For example, when the unit of analysis is a managerial function such as planning, the usefulness of the data is limited because of lack of information about the nature or object of the planning i.e., "Planning for what?" An approach which utilizes functional departments as the unit of analysis and specifies the proportion of executive time devoted to each fails to indicate the problem or responsibility demanding the executive's time. Coding problems likewise plague such approaches. Ambiguities occur in assigning executive activities to such overlapping categories as planning and control, and various organizations group different functions within departments having similar titles.

In our research, we assume that individual roles are a joint function of environmental, organizational, and individual influences. Such a view is an extension of "contingency" theories of organizations and leadership.[3] The nature of the role is dependent upon the situational context within which it occurs as well as the preferences and power of the role performer.

We view organizations as both a means of individuals using the organization in pursuit of individual goals and as a collectivity using individuals in pursuit of corporate objectives.[4] Exchanges between the organization and elements outside the organization provide part of the resources allocated in a series of internal exchanges to induce contributions from members. The nature of the product exchanged externally by the organization largely defines the character of the other external exchanges necessary for organizational functioning. For example, if the product exchanged is health care, the organization must engage in an intrinsically-related series of exchanges concerned with legal status (licensure), professional legitimacy (accreditation, certification), professional expertise (hiring certified health workers), etc. Levine and White list the three main categories of elements typically exchanged by health-related organizations:

1. referral of cases, clients, or patients;
2. giving or receiving of labor services encompassing the use of volunteers, lent personnel, and offering of instruction to personnel of other organizations, and
3. sending or receiving resources other than labor services, including funds, equipment, case and technical information.[5]

As we have said, to accomplish these exchanges, an organization must relate to elements outside itself in the environment. Duncan has divided the organization's external environment into five categories:

- customer component (distributors and users of product)
- supplier component (providers of labor, materials, equipment, and parts)
- competitor component (competitors for customers, suppliers)
- sociopolitical component (government regulators, public attitudes toward industry, organization product, and the relationship with trade unions)
- technological component (meeting new technological requirements of own industry and related industries and improving and developing new products by implementing new technological advances in the industry)[6]

Which of these environmental elements is relevant to an organization depends on how dependent the organization is on valued resources provided by the element, and on the strategies adopted by the organization to handle such dependencies. For example, the fact individuals rather than organizations are licensed to perform functions related to the healing arts makes delivery organizations particularly dependent upon professions and professionals. Faced with a dependency on professionals, an organization such as a hospital might adopt a strategy of employing physicians to alleviate this dependency. The ultimate strategy of managing dependence is to simply choose the product having the environment deemed most benevolent i.e., Weick's notion of chosen and enacted environments.[7]

Being an open system vulnerable to uncontrolled, often unpredictable environmental influences, organizations must assess relevant elements in their environment, predict their future probable states, select objectives, select strategies of controlling organizational activity toward such objectives, and monitor feedback of actual performance. The most general statement of the categories of organizational activities made necessary by the open systems perspective is that offered by Katz and Kahn.[8] These activities, which will be presented and discussed in detail later in the paper, are:

- adaptive subsystem activities to sense the environment and make recommendations for organizational response;
- boundary-spanning, production-supportive subsystem activities to negotiate with the environment, to secure resource inputs, and dispose of outputs;
- production subsystem activities concerned with producing the organization's principal product;
- maintenance subsystem activities concerned with maintaining the human and material resources and providing organizational stability;
- managerial subsystem activities to coordinate and control relations between functional departments and hierarchical levels and optimize relations between the organization and its environment.

The Katz and Kahn typology is useful in identifying the types of organizational activities required by open systems. However, knowing organizational activities is not the same as knowing the activities of a single role within an organization. To provide our explanation of the relationship between environmental and structural influences and executive role activities, we introduce Figure 1.

The principal outputs exchanged by delivery organizations are custody, diagnosis, treatment, referral, and sometimes research and education. (Figure 1, Box 1) Such outputs recommend appropriate technology, principal among which is medical technology. In one sense, physicians can be seen as being outside delivery organizations, presenting them with demands for certain types of services. Physicians could be viewed as the real "customers" or "salesmen" for such delivery organizations.[9] The nature of the physician's demands depends on the nature of the technology appropriate to his medical specialty. For example, the radiologist presents to hospitals the need for certain expensive equipment and trained personnel that differ from demands presented by the psychiatrist. Hence, our measure of technology is the

FIGURE 1

THEORETICAL PERSPECTIVE

Strategies of Control

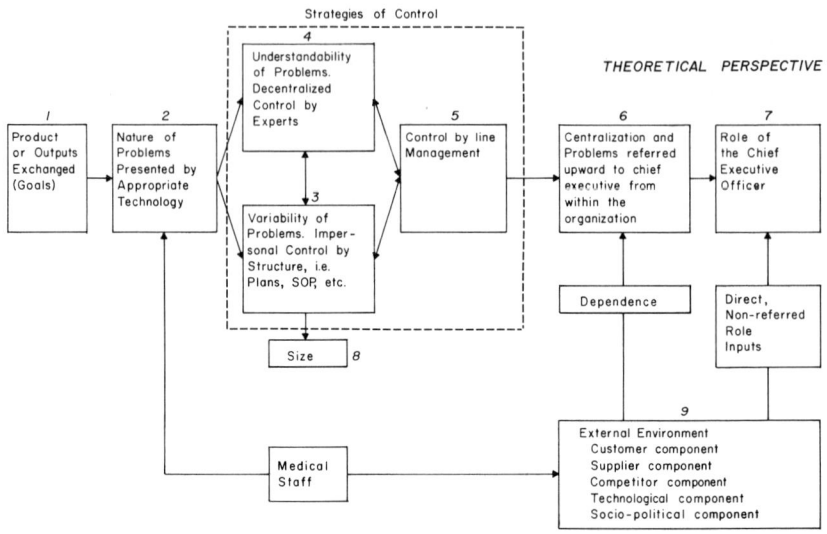

number of different medical specialties routinely admitting/serving patients in the organization.

What we have referred to as technology, the Aston group terms "operating variability" and Heydebrand terms "complexity of task structure."[10] We recognize that by measuring only the number of physician specialties, we have ignored the range of demands presented by general practice physicians. Since every delivery organization would be associated with at least one general practitioner, this scale item would have added little to the discriminatory power of the measure. Considering that GP's can call forth a wide range of technological responses on the part of a delivery organization, an organization having no specialists associated with it would still be characterized by a certain minimum level of technical complexity. This in fact is the case with LTC facilities. Due to the loose relationship between physicians and LTC facilities, we were unable to accurately determine the type of physician specialists associated with such organizations. Consequently, our measure produced a zero score rather than a low numerical value for LTC facilities. (Table 1, "Technology")

STRATEGIES OF CONTROL

As we have portrayed the concept here, technology exists separately and independently of any one delivery organization. Whether and how an organization responds to the demands of technology is an organizational choice. The essence of management is control of means toward desired ends. Managers choose among three broad "strategies of control" in their efforts to respond to the demands of technology and other external and internal influences. Perrow's model is helpful in identifying these strategies and their association with technology.[11]

Rather than deal with the descriptive, literal aspects of a given technology, Perrow takes a more cognitive approach by dealing with the nature of the search process involved in solving problems associated with the technology. Since the problem-solving process is inherently related to the nature of the raw material presenting the problems, he introduces a second variable he terms "variability" of raw materials. The interaction among these two variables in turn heavily influences the nature of the coordinative mechanism characterizing the task structure. Considering organizations as sociotechnical systems seeking predictability and control, each of these three variables may be seen

TABLE 1
STRUCTURAL CHARACTERISTICS OF HEALTH ORGANIZATIONS

Variable	Hospitals	Long-Term Care*	Medical Clinics	HMO's
Technology	19.3	0.0	12.5	18.5
Specialization	25.3	7.0	14.8	19.5
Expertise	32%	13%	28%	39%
Formalization	3.77	3.89	2.97	2.98
Dependence	62.8%	57.2%	0.00	2.3%**
Centralization	4.27	5.2	5.3	4.5

* All data for LTC are for individual facilities—excluding headquarters groups for the three facilities that are a part of a corporate chain. This makes a real difference in the matter of "expertise" since the relatively low expertise within the branch facility of a chain is offset considerably by the very high level of expertise available to them from their corporate headquarters. Expertise, using the present method, averages 42% for the three corporate headquarters offices. Specialization for central office only = 10.0

** Our measure of dependence: the proportion of funds deriving from third parties having ability to influence how the provider operated his facility (i.e., Blue Cross, Government) was inappropriate for HMO's since sometimes almost 100% of their funds derived from an external group having power to constrain, i.e., organized clientele, members.

as conscious strategies chosen by management to gain such predictability and control. Management chooses the value of each of these variables. Each strategy is an alternative method of control which is interdependent with the other two. Hence, to increase predictability, management can reduce the variability of the raw materials it processes, (i.e., a hospital can choose to treat only one class of illness such as female disorders or tuberculosis). Alternatively, an organization can continue to receive the same raw material inputs but increase predictability and control through increasing its ability to handle that type raw material i.e., increasing the ratio of specialists to primary-care physicians and/or introducing newer, more complex diagnostic-therapeutic equipment. Finally, greater control could be attempted through an increased emphasis on hierarchical control i.e., more, better, or more powerful line managers. The success in handling these strategies of control influences the number of cases or problems that are not handled well and therefore must be referred upward to the chief executive. As we see it, therefore, these three strategies of organizational control operate together to influence the problems and responsibilities referred up to the chief executive in delivery-type organizations. (Boxes 3 through 6 in Figure 1)

Control Through Reducing Variability—(Figure 1, Box 3)

The evidence of control is predictable results. It is evident that, *ceteris paribus,* the simpler the problem confronting the individual the greater the possibility of obtaining successful, predictable results in handling the problem. Hence, those management actions taken to reduce the difficulty and variability of problems presented to individuals for solution increase the level of control.

There are several strategies for reducing the variability and increasing the uniformity of raw materials or problems to be handled by individuals. First, the organization may simply choose to process a simpler class of raw materials or problems to be solved by the organization. When an LTC facility chooses to not admit mental patients, it simplifies its task complexity and avoids task demands that may lessen the predictability of results it presently enjoys. The same would be true of an HMO that chooses not to add psychiatric benefits to its benefits package. Second, an organization can fail to perceive the inherent variability of the raw materials it is already processing. Perrow makes it clear that his model addresses the perceived rather than the real nature of raw materials.[12] For example, behavioral scientists and nurses have long held that hospitals are "curing" physical ailments of bodily organs and processes rather than "caring" for the entire range of psychosocial-physiological problems that could be handled by a more holistic approach to patients as humans.[13] Clearly, the work of health organizations would be significantly more complex, and the level of predictability lower if they addressed all the causes of physical and psychological pathology among their patient populations!

A third strategy for reducing variability of raw material inputs is to reduce the range and difficulty of problems confronting an individual by dividing the task among several positions. Technology presents a solution to a complete problem. It is management's choice as to whether and to what extent that problem shall be solved by individuals or groups. Maytag chooses to let one worker construct an entire washing machine while other manufacturers choose to divide this task among many workers on an assembly line. How to make a machine or solve a patient's problem is a question of "machine technology." How such a solution is implemented within an organization is a managerial decision based on "administrative technology."[14] Machine technology specifies only the complete set of necessary procedures while administrative technology recommends how the set of procedures shall be divided into subsets i.e., functional specialization.

In our study, we measured functional specialization along an ordinal scale of 1 to 39 representing different "functional specialisms" adapted by the research group from a smaller scale developed by the Aston Group.[15] Each scale point is a type of work rather than an occupational title—thus avoiding the problem of having similar titles for dissimilar duties. It could be expected that the more varied the task demands placed on organizations by technology, the greater the functional specialization within organizations to reduce this complexity—a relationship which in fact obtained in the organizations we studied. (Table 1)

A fourth method of reducing the variability associated with handling raw materials is through specification of standard procedures and rules. In our research, we operationalized this variable by use of a Guttman-type scale incorporating the extent to which standard procedures have been developed, extent to which such procedures have been officially recognized, and extent to which such official and standard procedures are in fact adhered to in practice. (Table 1, "Formalization")

The four methods of reducing variability appear often in the literature under a variety of titles. Three of the dimensions of Bureaucracy specified by Weber and operationalized by Hall serve a similar purpose (i.e., division of labor, rules, and procedures).[16] The first factor extracted in the statistical analysis by the Aston Group and termed "structuring of activities" contains specialization, standardization, formalization, and concentration of authority. This last item is similar to our third strategy of control. Their inclusion of it in the same factor along with items similar to our first strategy is not inconsistent considering the negative loading of the former and the positive loadings of the latter.[17] Reliance on both specialization and formalization is referred to by March and Simon as "coordination by plan."[18] All of these methods relate to externalized, impersonalized means of management control that is sometimes so subtle that it is hardly perceived as such by subordinates.[19] It may be impersonal in nature, but it is nonetheless a quite effective strategy of control. Rules and procedures are more palatable than verbal commands.

Control Through Increasing Understandability
(Figure 1, Box 4)

The simplest way to process raw materials is by hiring individuals possessing the skills appropriate to the class of decisions involved in handling that type raw material. Clearly, the predictability of the organization's performance increases as the proportion of individuals with the appropriate expertise increases. Hence, a non-bureaucratic mode of organization control is through self and collegial control associated with the expertise of employees. A related form of control is the expertise incorporated into machines.

Control through expertise is constrained by the nature of the technological demands placed on the organization. For example, the technology of surgery is much better understood than that of the mind. It would be possible to array the various medical specialties along a continuum of uncertainty.[20] Specialties characterized by relatively high levels of certainty and predictability would *permit* lower levels of expertise although legal barriers and professional self-interests would militate against organizations employing non-professionals to perform such tasks. Hence, there is an inherent relationship between the range and degree of uncertainty characterizing the technology placing demands on the organization and the level of employee expertise needed to properly handle such task demands——a relationship born out by our measures. (Table 1)

In our research, we measured Expertise as the proportion of employees earning as much or more than the entry-level, inexperienced registered nurse in that organization. The assumption was that this position requires a somewhat standard level of professional preparation and expertise which would be reflected in the pay for that position. It was assumed that similar levels of expertise among other positions would be accurately reflected in pay levels for those positions. Hence, employees earning as much or more than the beginning RN were presumed to have as much or more expertise than the RN. A score of 39 percent for HMO's is taken to mean that this proportion of employees has expertise comparable to the R.N. (Table 1) Since the measure excludes physicians, it undervalues the expertise available to organizations having physicians working for them on a continuing basis. Adding physicians to the expertise measure for clinics raises it from 28 to 39 percent; for HMO's the figure increases from 39 to 47 percent. The presence of such an expert group of employees who, in the case of physicians, is also an organized and powerful group, certainly leads to greater reliance on self and collegial control and lessened reliance on procedural and hierarchical forms of control—a phenomenon that in fact obtained in clinics and HMO's as we shall discuss later in the paper.

This strategy of control appears in the literature under a variety of titles. It is the third factor extracted in the statistical analysis of the Aston Group and termed "line control of workflow" i.e., control resting in the hands of workflow personnel themselves, and well-developed personnel procedures for selecting employees qualified to make such decisions.[21] Hage and Aiken utilize a similar measure they call "degree of complexity."[22] Building on Litwak's work, Hall found professionalization and bureaucratization to be inversely correlated to each other and related to the degree of routine involved in task performance.[23] Montagna reports in his study of a large accounting firm that where procedures were routinized, computers replaced experts.[24] Note that this merely shifts the source of expertise from humans to equipment rather than from expertise to some alternative strategy of control.[25] Hickson refers to this concept as "knowledge technology."[26] Perrow's concept of "understandability" and most of the other authors cited here refer back to an earlier distinction between "algorithmic" and "heuristic" problems made by Simon et al.[27] Problems solvable through determinate search procedures are intrinsically simpler and capable of being handled through delegation to groups of lesser-trained individuals than the heuristic-type problems requiring problemistic, nondeterminate search procedures i.e., intuition informed by extensive knowledge. Some feel multi-part problems are simpler and lend themselves better to solution by delegation to groups than the more difficult multi-stage problems best solved by individuals.[28] While the terms and usage vary among authors writing in this field of inquiry, they are referring to essentially the same concept we have addressed as "understandability" and expertise as a strategy of control.

CONTROL BY MANAGERS— (Figure 1, Box 5)

According to Perrow, the interaction between understandability and variability is hypothesized to influence the task structure. Low variability of raw materials plus high understandability in how to process such materials should be associated with bureaucratic structure i.e., coordination by plan. Conversely, highly variable raw materials and low understandability of how to deal with problems presented by such materials should be associated with control by feedback and collaboration such as characterizes collegial, professional-type organizations.[29] As we have said, the Aston Group found centralization of authority negatively correlated with other items in their "structuring of activities" dimension.[30] The issue involved is the relationship between control by managerial decision and such alternative forms of control as impersonalized structure and expertise.

In our research, we operationalized hierarchical control by use of the "concentration of authority" measure used by the Aston Group.[31] Their measure identifies the average *level* at which a group of typical decisions are made. This does not identify the positions or role involved. However, since in our study the higher the level the closer the locus of decision is to the highest role in the organization, the measure provides an indication of the tendency for decisions to be made by the role we were studying. Hence, though it is a measure intended for use where the organization is the unit of analysis, it was deemed appropriate for use where the unit of analysis is the highest-level role. The measure varies in value from 1 for the scale-point representing the non-managerial operative employee to 6 for the Board of Control. Scale point 5 is the chief executive officer. Based on the group of decisions used with this scale in our study, these organizations are fairly centralized, (Table 1).

To this point, we have developed the theory and methodology of the relationship between strategies of organizational control and the number of exceptional cases referred to the chief executive officer for decision. (Figure 1, Boxes 1 through 6) The nature of the crucial problems and responsibilities handled by the chief executive (Figure 1,

Box 7) would depend not only on how technology was thus handled through various strategies of control but as well on the operation of other, non-technical, environmental variables.

ENVIRONMENTAL INFLUENCES ON ROLES—Figure 1, Box 9)

There appears to be an inverse relation between dependence on the environment and centralization of decision making. It is well known that unionization within a company removes much of the power of making personnel policies from the foremen and centralizes it.[32] Relations between the organization and the external union on which it depends so importantly are too crucial to be settled ad hoc and inconsistently at the foreman level. Similarly, the dependence of health service delivery organizations on physicians makes physician recruitment and medical staff relations a matter for concern by the highest levels of decision within such organizations. Hence, it is understandable that organizational dependence is positively correlated with centralization of the class of decision related to such dependence.[33]

In our study, our direct measure of organizational dependence is the proportion of organization revenues coming from third parties having the power to constrain the organization's operations. That is, how financially dependent is the organization on third party payors whose funds have strings attached, i.e., Blue Cross, Medicare, Medicaid. This measure failed to produce a meaningful measure of dependence for HMO's since their funds originate entirely from members' dues, (Table 1). Where such members are organized and exercising influence over organizational affairs, a better measure might be one related to such consumer influence. Where members are unorganized as in the foundation for medical care-type HMO, it could be there is in fact little dependence on consumers—such HMO's are perhaps as financially independent of consumers as clinics are presently, (Table 1). While we measured only financial dependence, clearly there are many forms of dependence on environmental elements that influence centralization of decision making. In our analysis, we shall refer to organizational dependence on most of the environmental categories alluded to in Box 9, Figure 1.

In this section we have been developing our theoretical perspective of the relation between environment, organization structure, and the executive role, (Figure 1). In addition, we have given our operational measures of the key variables involved, (Table 1). It should be stressed that this contingency view is a theory of how an organizational environment affects an organization. Since it does not hypothesize any one best way of characterizing groups of organizations, grouped data such as are in Table 1 are less illustrative of the theory than would be data for an individual organization. In the role analysis to follow, therefore, we shall rely less on the quantitative data in Table 1 than on qualitative information about the variables recommended by the theory. That is, the usefulness of the perspective is in identifying the relevant variables to examine and to provide insights into the relationship among variables. The theory proved to be very useful in doing this in this exploratory study. In a definitive study involving a larger sample size it would be possible to make explicit use of quantitative measures of each of the variables in the analysis.

Having provided this theoretical background on the perspective guiding the collection and analysis of data, we turn now to an explanation of the variable of interest in the study, the role of the health service administrator.

Method

Using a perspective in which it is held that executive activities flow from and are a subject of organizational activities, it becomes necessary to specify first the organization activities and from that derive the role activities of the executive. In the previous section we discussed a theory of how organization activities become role activities. In this section we shall provide a methodology for specifying organizational and role activities.

As we have said, in our approach we view the executive role as flowing primarily from organizational activities. This requires a typology of required organizational activities within delivery organizations as viewed from a social system perspective. Our approach begins with the Katz and Kahn model which specifies the five organization sub-systems listed in Table 2.[34] Since these categories specify only the broadest of activity types, it was necessary to specify the individual organizational activities within each of the five subsystems. We began with the list of sixteen generic, staff-like organizational "specialisms" the Aston Group developed from an earlier paper by Bakke.[35] To these were added managerial and line-type production activities specific to health service delivery organizations. Some of these activities were from the Aston Group's "centralization" index. The result was a Standard List of 46 Organizational Activities. The items were general enough to be useful with all levels of employees in all types of health service delivery organizations yet specific enough to provide insights into the nature of role activity.

Two scales were used to allow respondents to indicate which of the 46 organizational activities were relevant to their roles. Respondents indicated both their degree and type of personal involvement in each of the activities and the importance of the activity to their role. Combining these importance and involvement scores allowed identification of the approximately 40 percent of the organizational activities which were "crucial" role activities. Those role activities which are crucial to each type executive are marked by an "X" in Table 2.

To test our assignment of these activities to the five sub-system categories of Katz and Kahn, six Ph.D. candidates in Organizational Psy-

TABLE 2
Taxonomy of Organizational Activities

I. Adaptive Subsystem Activities:
Oriented toward external environment. Intelligence, research, development, planning activities resulting in *recommendations* to managerial subsystem for purpose of assiting organization in changing, adapting, surviving.

Activity	Hosp.	LTC	Clinic	HMO	Activity
1.	X		X	X	Market research
2.	X		X		Product research
31.	X	X	X	X	Long-range planning
	3	1	3	2	

II. Supportive/Boundary Subsystem Activities:
Carries out two types of exchanges between organization and elements within organization's external environment: (1) securing production-related inputs of materials and manpower and disposing of outputs; (2) legitimating the organization through image building and manipulation of relevant elements in organization's environment.

Activity	Hosp.	LTC	Clinic	HMO	Activity
3.	X	X	X	X	Public Relations
4.	X	X		X	Lobbying: influencing rulings of gov't. agencies
7.		X			Determine buying procedures
10.	X			X	Obtaining long-term capital
11.			X		Obtaining working capital; collections
14.		X		X	Labor negotiations
15.	X	X		X	Establish agreements with other health organizations
20.					Decisions re: appointments of physicians
22.	X	X	X	X	Recruiting professionals, physicians
46.	X			X	Negotiating with powerful external org's.
	6	6	3	7	

III. Production Subsystem Activities:

Activities related to accomplishing the most directly goal-related tasks. Throughput activities re: transforming information, materials, people, etc.

Activity	Hosp.	LTC	Clinic	HMO	Activity
6.					Transporting, distributing patients, supplies
19.					Decisions re: patient appointments, routing, etc.
36.					Decisions re: nursing care given
37.		X			Decisions re: dietary services, patient food
38.					Decisions re: laundry and linen
39.					Decisions re: medical-type records
40.				X	Decisions re: housekeeping
41.					Decisions re: diagnosis of patients i.e., x-ray, lab, etc.
42.					Decisions re: treatment of patients i.e., medical and nursing orders, drugs, therapy, P.T., O.T., etc.
	0	1	0	1	

IV. Maintenance Subsystem Activities:

Mediating between demands of the tasks and needs of the members to achieve greater predictability, stability. Concerned with both the human and material "equipment" necessary for work. Socializing members; setting up reward systems and monitoring performance; standardizing and formalizing procedures ("SOP"), etc.

Activity	Hosp.	LTC	Clinic	HMO	Activity
9.	X	X	X	X	Decisions re: professional/managerial salaries
17.		X	X		Devising work procedures for professionals
18.			X		Devising work procedures for nonprofessionals
21.	X	X	X	X	Promoting/rewarding professionals/managers
23.					Routine work assignment scheduling
24.		X	X		Employee/management development and training
25.		X			Disciplining professional/managerial employees
27.		X			Decisions re: maintaining building/equipment
32.	X	X	X	X	Motivating directing immediate subordinates
35.					Disciplining/dismissing physicians
43.	X	X	X	X	Dealing with personal/interpersonal problems
	4	8	7	4	

V. Managerial Subsystem Activities:

Though defined as a "sub" system, actually closer to a "supra" system having activities that cut across, overlay other four subsystems. Purposes are: (1) control = resolving conflicts between hierarchical levels; (2) coordination = optimizing relations between functional (horizontal) substructures, adjudicating between them; (3) optimizing relations between organization and environment, deciding whether and how to implement recommendations of adaptive subsystem (the implementation being carried out by supportive subsystem, however).

Activity	Hosp.	LTC	Clinic	HMO	Activity
5.		X	X		Decisions re: charges/prices for services etc.
8.					Decisions re: type new equipment needed
12.					Approving exceptions to budget of less than $500.
13.					Determine cost finding system or items to be studied
16.	X	X		X	Developing criteria/systems to control quality
26.	X	X	X	X	Decisions re: new construction
28.			X	X	Creating/changing professional job/units
29.	X	X	X	X	Decisions re: changes in decision/authority structure
30.	X	X	X	X	Decisions re: financial/managerial information system
33.	X	X	X	X	Influencing decisions of Board/Owners
34.	X		X	X	Influencing decisions made by Medical Staff
44.			X	X	Arbitrate between internal units, departments
45.	X		X	X	Arbitrate between policy-making groups
	7	6	9	9	

chology from the Institute of Social Research at the University of Michigan were asked to replicate our judgments. The Institute is the employing organization of Professors Katz and Kahn. Statistical analysis of the degree of consensus among independent ratings by these individuals produced a "kappa" value indicating overall agreement 40 percent in excess of that which could be expected to have occurred by chance alone. (Standard Error .062) [36] Tests of their agreement with the choices we made as shown in Table 2 indicated agreement 59 percent in excess of chance.[37]

Use of the term "standard" list does not imply the activities are in any way standardized or routine. Standard means simply a single or common list of organizational activities developed on an a priori basis. The advantage of this approach is the ability to compare the variation in responses to a single stimulus—a necessity in comparative research. The disadvantage of this approach is the failure to anticipate all relevant activities on an a priori bases. To overcome this deficiency, we developed a complementary set of open-ended questions in which the subsystem category was given to the respondent as a cue or probe. He was asked to volunteer any "crucial responsibilities and problems" he might have that are logically related to that general class of organizational activity. While the results of that approach are not presented here, the analysis presented here did involve reference to such responses. In general, this free response mode produced few types of activities not anticipated in the Standard List, but it did provide the richness of detail missing in the more structured approach. Complementing the field research was an extensive review of the literature in each of the relevant areas of theory and research. Draft copies of the analysis were shared with a subset of the respondents to verify our preliminary conclusions.

Two approaches were used to provide insight into the question of the relationship between these role activities and educational preparation. The first approach involved respondents scoring each item in the Standard List according to the best source of obtaining competence to perform the activity. Nine response categories were provided ranging from inherited attributes to a professional degree program. Responses were aggregated into three categories i.e., "other," "self," and "educational institution." The second approach involved the direct question of indicating which five of the 46 activities respondents feel health administration programs should stress.

Results: The Role of the Health Services Administrator

Of the "crucial" role activities (indicated by an "X" in Table 2), 17 are crucial to three or four of the roles. An additional 13 activities are not considered crucial to any of the four roles. These 30 activities comprise the major points of commonality between these four roles. The remaining 16 items are activities that are unique to only one or two of the roles—providing many of the points of difference among the roles. The hospital role is the most generic in that it is characterized by all 17 common core role activities common to three or four of the roles and is not characterized by any activity unique to itself. The LTC role is the least generic of the roles studied in that it is characterized by fewer of the common core activities and contains the most unique activities. The hospital and HMO executive roles are quite similar. The medical group manager role falls between the hospital and HMO roles on the one hand and LTC executives on the other.

Clearly, there is a great deal of commonality among these roles.

These similarities occurring as they do among executives within a single sector of the same industry lends some support to the hypothesized relations between technology and organization structure as they ultimately influence role activities. Since chief executives are one or more hierarchical levels removed from activity differences introduced by technology, our focus on a single role at the apex of the organization likewise tended to produce role similarities. That is, a study of the highest-level role removes the differences inherit in the "machine technology" employed at operating levels in the organization and documents the generic nature of the "administrative technology" common across organizations at this hierarchical level. Although the terminology and method of aggregating discrete activities differs, the common core activities identified in our study are quite consistent with those identified by Mintzberg in his recent study.[38] At a certain level of abstraction, there do appear to be certain universal managerial activities.[39] Empirical studies tend to support the following conclusions about managerial roles: (1) an emphasis on planning or structuring the decision environment for others as contrasted to performing or supervising performance; (2) tend to deal with less structured situations and problems having longer, more futuristic time frames; (3) greater orientation toward external environment than internal affairs.[40] Since ours was an exploratory study designed to answer other questions, we cannot go beyond saying our data are consistent with these conclusions from other studies.

Adopting the convention that the common core activities characterizing three or more roles represent a tentative description of the role of the health service administrator, we shall examine that role as it relates to each of the five organizational subsystems, (Table 2). We shall, of course, also be comparing the four roles studied in the research.

The data reveal a relatively great concern with adaptive type activities such as market and product research, and long-range planning. In an industry characterized by monopoly, one naturally wonders why executives would be motivated to engage in activities focused on organizational flexibility and survival. LTC executives are not concentrating on such activities because their heavy reliance on federal funds creates a dependence on federal guidelines for programs. In effect, LTC executives are reacting to external imperatives more than they are sensing market conditions and initiating change.[41] Chain-type LTC corporations engage in a great deal of forward planning at the corporate level, but it is done by staff specialists more than by the chief operating executives we interviewed. The motivations are presumably similar to those of executives of public utilities where it is necessary to react to edicts of the public utility commission.

It would be erroneous to equate the "research" activities of these executives with the view of research activities advocated in college courses drawn from experiences in profit-oriented, product-type industries. To Procter and Gamble, "market" means the consuming public. While the public is the ultimate consumer of medical services, it is mostly in the "co-op" type HMO's that executives are engaged in anything resembling classic market and product research. In the other types of organizations, executives are vitally concerned with marketing, but they define the market as the "principal sources of resources." Since physicians provide patients to these organizations, physicians are in fact the operational definition of the market for these organizations. "Research" in this case means such activities as: (1) keeping up with trends in medicine and the types of services offered in their size and type of facility, (2) efforts to attract adequate numbers and types of physicians, (3) knowing the competition, and (4) knowing changes in politics of funding and regulatory agencies. Product research may be as casual as emulating the competition or some role-model facility reported in the industry's trade journal, or buying some new technology introduced to the organization by a salesman. Often it is the lay executive who then sells the medical staff on the equipment or service rather than the medical staff selling the administration. An exception is the HMO where the Medical Staff has both the financial incentive and a group structure enabling them to take initiatives in the area of product research. What is clear is that the executives we studied are not researching the health needs of the population as is taught in consumer-oriented research commonly taught in college courses. In contrast to the traditional focus in research on consumer characteristics on the demand side, health service organizations enjoying a relatively high degree of monopoly power tend to focus on research of factors related to providers of care on the supply side.

Everyone "sells," only the definitions differ. As long as social organizations are open systems vulnerable to uncontrolled inputs and constraints from their environment, boundary-spanning transactions with such groups will be necessary. Such exchanges go under names like public relations, negotiations, lobbying, recruiting, contracting, etc. It may be significant that clinics, the organizations with the most monopoly power of those we studied, were the least involved in such activities. By our measures, they scored zero (0) in "dependence," (Table 1).

The health service administrator is engaged in seeking legitimization for himself and his organization through speeches and service in various groups in the community. Heavy dependence on federal and state funds and regulations causes all but the clinic manager to engage in influencing legislation and rulings of pertinent agencies of federal and state governments. This may mean literally lobbying in the direct sense, calling one's local legislator, or calling the executive director of their trade association. In the smaller organizations—LTC facilities and clinics—executives were directly involved in relations with the consuming public. Since family members actually make the decision to admit the elderly to LTC facilities, LTC administrators are continually engaged in currying the favor of individuals who have or might admit patients. An announced goal of LTC facilities is to increase the proportion of patients who pay for their own care i.e., private-pay patients. In the early stages of growth where reaching the financial break-even point is crucial, marketing aimed at employed groups is a crucial concern of HMO executives.

Chief executives are quite involved in almost every type of exchange their respective organizations engage in. They are quite attuned to those aspects of their environment crucial to organizational survival and growth. Whether it is making agreements with related health organizations, negotiating with the local planning agency, state regulatory agency, accrediting group, city planner, or labor union, these executives are quite involved. However, their most crucial activity both in terms of importance and time, is probably that of recruiting key professionals and physicians. As we have said, the real market is the physician who admits patients and the real producer is a set of key physicians for whom legally there are no substitutes. Unlike other industries where management's efforts can increase sales and provide adequately trained employees, these decisions are largely uncontrollable by health service executives. Hence, they must recruit. Especially in the larger hospitals, they may try to close the system by entering into contractual arrangements to provide house staff physicians.

To better control the supply of other key professionals, the organization can begin its own training program, encourage the local community college to begin such a program, or substitute lesser-trained individuals.

It is clear from observation of the *Production Subsystem* (Table 2) the health service administrator is not directly involved in such activities. Our data match well the conceptualizations of Thompson who sees the "technological core" as the most closed part of the organization and of Simon et al who view the role of management as closing this part of the organization by structuring the decisional environment. Hence, although executives aren't directly involved in either performing or supervising performance of the highly technical work of providing diagnosis, cure, and custody of patients, they are indirectly working to ensure that such services are routinized and rationalized. Lack of technical expertise by lay executives and legal prohibitions against laymen making medical decisions have given rise to the very real phenomenon of the dual hierarchy in which physicians and other professionals dominate the delivery subsystem within health organizations. However, while this militates against personal involvement and interpersonal forms of influence by the lay executive, it does not preclude the less obvious but no less effective forms of impersonal influence i.e., defining scope of services, programming, standardizing, recruiting, etc. The health service administrators is involved, but more in the sense that the late Henry Ford still influences those who work on the assembly line he popularized over a half century ago. In theoretical terms, control is more by experts and structure and less by hierarchical control.

The most obvious feature of the *Maintenance Subsystem* (Table 2) is how emphasis on these types of activities varies inversely with size of organization. Executives in LTC facilities and clinics, both of which organizations average about 100 employees, are more concerned with such activities than executives in the larger hospitals and HMO's. Even so, all these executives are personally involved in decisions concerning salaries and promotions of key individuals, motivating their key subordinates, and handling personal and interpersonal problems of key individuals.

The health service administrator especially in larger facilities, is normally dealing primarily with his subordinates and others who occupy key positions of influence. Even though executives in the larger organizations are engaged in fewer maintenance-type activities, our research design does not permit the conclusion that this class of activities is less important than activities in other subsystems. It is still true in large organizations that employee-centered, group-process type activities are necessary concomitants of production or task-centered activities. Whereas task and process leader roles may well be held by different individuals in the larger organizations, in LTC facilities and clinics chief executives must give attention to both roles. Of all the roles studied, the medical group manager is most involved in group maintenance activities. Since his is the task of, in effect, managing his superiors, he must possess either the ability to acquiesce to their desires or superior ability to influence them toward his managerial initiatives. We turn now to an examination of the essence of the managerial role i.e., the managerial subsystem.

With the exception of LTC, the emphasis on *Managerial Subsystem* activities is relatively equal among the organizations studied, (Table 2). Differences in the LTC role arise from two structural features i.e., monolithic power structure and lack of an organized medical staff. Of course, it is the presence of an organized medical staff in delivery organizations that makes their power structure pluralistic in nature. LTC facilities are typically privately owned and controlled by either the owner or his agent. While LTC facilities are required to have physicians visit patients and perform certain functions required by the government, this provides physicians little leverage over owners of the facilities. Since such physicians serve at the pleasure of the owner of the LTC facility, physicians lack a base of power from which they might effectively countervail the power of the owners. Hence, the LTC executive is not engaged in negotiating between policy-making groups or between semi-autonomous professional departments.

The essence of organization and therefore the principal role of management is control. Organizations seek to order reality toward some idealized state or collective level of aspiration. At the most general level of abstraction, management activities involve prognostication and planning of the ideal or hoped-for state of reality, devising of methods and measures of acceptable progress toward the goal, collection of feedback or information about actual performance, and the taking of corrective action. Some of these control activities have already been discussed under the other four subsystems. Three of the activities fall within the managerial subsystem.

First, the health service administrator is engaged in activities concerning the authority structure making the decisions i.e., influencing decisions by the owners or Board of Control. The medical group manager presents an interesting example of the problem presented in these types of activities. He has a task similar to that of leaders in voluntary organizations who must first elicit the consent of the governed before they can govern. He must "manipulate" his superiors to gain the legitimacy and base of authority necessary to "manage" his subordinates.[42] To do this, he influences whether and to what extent the physician-owners organize, who gets appointed to what positions within the resulting structure, what issues are placed on the agenda, and what fact sets they use in deciding. Notice that he is not passively waiting for them to do these things; he is influencing these processes. Contrary to classic management theory, the manager is manipulating the owners through reliance on bases of power other than legitimate authority.[43]

The hospital administrator has a somewhat different problem. Medical staffs in hospitals must organize, therefore the hospital administrator is concerned with managing their exercise of power. He must encourage them to organize yet keep them from using their power to actually run the hospital. As one administrator put it, he must guide their use of power to a position of planned responsibility midway between the extremes of uninvolvement and assertion. Translated, this means manipulating the type and degree of their participation in decision making.

Having influenced whether and how boards and medical staffs organize, the health service administrator influences which matters are brought before such groups for decision (agenda building) and how such issues are decided. The biggest such decision in health service organizations relates to the criteria of quality employed in judging the services provided. In LTC facilities, these criteria originate largely from governmental agencies and are enforced through the monolithic power structure characterizing that type organization. In clinics, the owner-operators are the task group leaders providing the bulk of the services. Therefore, the clinic manager has little role in developing such quality control criteria. Since hospitals are increasingly being made responsible for the quality of care provided by the medical staff, to fulfill this responsibility hospital administrators are increasingly faced with the task of gaining sufficient authority over medical staffs. And, as we have seen, gaining such control in the absence of a sufficient formal base of power requires administrators to resort to manipulative strategies. The more ideal situation among those we studied exists within the HMO.

The structural feature of HMO's whereby both management and the medical staff are committed to a fixed, prospective budget provides a common fate tending to encourage the two groups to assume a problem solving rather than a negotiating posture toward each other. This non-zero sum distribution of outcomes leads to attitudes and behaviors better characterized as cooperation than as conflict. While pluralistic centers of power remain, the mode of interaction shifts from manipulation and bargaining to sharing of information and reliance on less coercive forms of interpersonal influence. Both the medical staff and administration are equally interested in usage patterns since both are constrained by an unyielding fixed sum of member revenues.

The inability to separate the responsibility of management and medical staff in the HMO leads to an unwillingness and in fact inability to separate their respective spheres of authority. The HMO executive and chief medical officer in effect exercise mutual veto power over each other. They have what Burns and Stalker refer to as a "rationale for non-definition" resulting in a purposive avoidance of clear lines of authority and function.[44] Only one-half the HMO executives had job descriptions and these considered them quite unrealistic representations of reality.

We have to this point discussed such aspects of control as authority structure, decision making, and specification of criteria. We have seen the variety of approaches each of the four executives takes to these common managerial tasks. They are all engaged in decisions concerning the management information system required to monitor performance. While it is true, especially in the larger organizations, that such monitoring is on the basis of a formal and written system of feedback, it is certainly not confined to that means. Executives in even the largest organizations engage in personal, informal monitoring which might be characterized as a sort of inspection tour. A useful metaphor for this approach might be the practice of Air Force pilots in which they search for "targets of opportunity" after they have fulfilled their assigned bombing run. Similarly, the health service administrator compares the visual reality about him with his personal and largely intuitive standards of quality. Such a tour might be no more than walking through the building and calling the executive housekeeper to report a dirty hallway, etc. While such is not the stuff of which college courses are made, it is very much a part of the essence of health service administration.

Katz and Kahn include within the managerial subsystem the general function of "optimizing relations between the organization and its environment." The crucial question in this function is the decision criterion used in the optimizing. That is, does the organization act in its own best interest in making a decision or act to optimize the health system? If a hospital is chronically full while neighboring hospitals are well below capacity, does the hospital build or encourage physicians to utilize other hospitals? Stated differently, does optimizing involve global or local rationality?[45] Does the chief executive officer guide policy making groups toward a set of internal decision criteria or stress a social welfare criterion?

In the sense that the health service administrator tries to get units within his organization to decide issues on the basis of what is good for the whole organization, he is encouraging "global rationality."

However, when dealing with issues whereby his organization stands to lose what is gained by other organizations, he exercises a "local rationality." It was clear from the free response questions in the structured interviews that these executives were not overly enamored with comprehensive health planning. Relations with neighboring health facilities of a similar type were perhaps superficially friendly, but the underlying posture was nonetheless that of competition. Optimizing in the case of one clinic faced by an equally powerful clinic nearby and a hospital threatening to enter into ambulatory care meant merger of the clinics to better equip them for facing the threat posed by the hospital. Optimizing for a hospital meant expanding into ambulatory care to counter the threat posed by proliferating group practices. Optimizing for the nursing home chain means allocating resources among the various branch facilities according to corporate-level global criteria of rationality.

This emphasis on internal, local criteria says more about our theories than it does about these organizations. Theorists can't have it both ways i.e., define groups and organizations on the basis of shared values and goals while advocating they act on behalf of the values and goals of outsiders. These executives acted on behalf of their organizations because they must. If they are to act differently, then these organizations must first be structurally integrated with the organizations with whom it is desired they act cooperatively. An example of this structural means of inducing global rationality would be the integrating function served by the prospective budget in the HMO by which common responsibility induced common authority.

Another means of encouraging decisions that put the system's interests ahead of the organization's would be professional status for executives. The physician can put the patient's interests ahead of the hospital's because only physicians can legally practice medicine and every physician has a medical staff and a profession to back his claim's to autonomy. The administrator has no legal protection and no professional group capable of successfully backing him. Consequently, he lacks the base of power necessary to be socially responsible. It is this deficiency that above all defeats the claims of executives to professional status.[46]

Educational Implications

In addition to collecting data on role content, we asked for other information bearing more directly on the question of educational preparation to perform role functions. Rather than directly assessing the knowledge and skills necessary to perform each of the role activities listed in Table 2, we asked respondents to indicate for each of these activities the best source of obtaining competence to perform the activity.

It is abundantly clear in Table 3 that these successful executives generally prefer "self" as the best source of obtaining requisite skills for their position. We could say this means either they have forgotten where they in fact learned their role skills, or they had poor educational preparation and learned mostly by experience. Or, we could say that the skills necessary for the chief executive are either not teachable or weren't taught to these respondents. One is always on firm ground in taking respondents at their word and assuming they in fact know what they are saying. These respondents are saying experience has been their best teacher.

How can we reconcile a complex role in a highly complex, technical organization with statements from some of the best leaders of such organizations to the effect that for them education is not the best way to prepare to perform their role? A possible answer might be that technical knowledge and discrete job skills—the emphasis of all graduate educational programs—simply are not the crucial variables for this role. It may well be as C. Wright Mills says, more a question of personal values and who you know than specialized knowledge such as middle-level managers must possess.[47] If it is matter of values, whose values? The chief executive probably must conform to the values of those who are "significant" to him either in terms of granting or withholding personal rewards or in being instrumental in aiding or blocking the decision process. As we have seen, he is most concerned with managing environmental dependence and internal decision making. Hence, the health service administrator could be expected to adopt the values of the power elites with whom he works, in and outside the organization. Tagiuri's study of executives, scientists, and research managers revealed research managers had value orientations consistent with their organizational positions.[48] That is, research managers were the "men in the middle" between scientists and executives. Research managers were found to have value sets representing an amalgam of the two groups with whom they worked. It is unlikely that it could be otherwise, for prolonged interaction between individuals with incompatible values and attitudes should result in either continual psychological or social conflict or changes in the conflicting values.

We did not directly assess executive values and attitudes or attempt to document the individuals and groups who would constitute the

TABLE 3
Source of Competence

Activity No.	Others	Self	Education	Activity No.	Others	Self	Education
1.	33%	43%	24%	24.	26%	37%	37%
2.	45%	41%	14%	25.	21%	71%	8%
3.	6%	71%	23%	26.	33%	54%	13%
4.	18%	64%	18%	27.	31%	57%	12%
5.	33%	78%	9%	28.	30%	44%	26%
6.	36%	52%	12%	29.	24%	46%	30%
7.	31%	49%	21%	30.	25%	42%	33%
8.	42%	52%	6%	31.	20%	54%	26%
9.	33%	57%	10%	32.	6%	73%	21%
10.	30%	46%	24%	33.	9%	71%	20%
11.	32%	45%	23%	34.	25%	57%	18%
12.	34%	64%	2%	35.	23%	69%	8%
13.	32%	38%	30%	36.	39%	42%	19%
14.	23%	48%	29%	37.	40%	40%	20%
15.	13%	63%	24%	38.	36%	45%	19%
16.	39%	22%	39%	39.	39%	33%	28%
17.	30%	44%	26%	40.	31%	50%	19%
18.	27%	44%	29%	41.	46%	27%	27%
19.	31%	48%	21%	42.	46%	29%	25%
20.	24%	65%	11%	43.	12%	76%	12%
21.	23%	67%	10%	44.	12%	78%	10%
22.	26%	61%	13%	45.	16%	61%	23%
23.	32%	57%	11%	46.	7%	71%	22%

Each respondent indicated both a first and a second choice for each of the activities in the Standard List of Activities, choices indicating the best and next best sources of obtaining the competence required to perform the activity. The above data are an average of both choices combined for the entire sample of respondents. (N=48 Max.)

Others: 1. Rely on others i.e., consult with other managers, staff experts, M.D.'s etc.

Self: 2. Personality, charm, persuasive and interpersonal skills.
3. Basic inherited intelligence; common sense.
4. Experience
5. Self-instruction, and read books, journal articles, etc.

Education: 6. A course, workshop, institute, etc., on a specific subject; continuing education.
7. Well-rounded, broad, general or liberal education.
8. Professional, specialized education.

set of significant others for these executives. A study incorporating these objectives is now underway. It is clear, however, that role incorporates these psychological attributes as well as role behaviors.[49] When executives indicate that experience, other forms of self preparation, and relying on others are more crucial than classroom instruction, they may well be telling us that these are the relevant arenas in which to gain personal attributes such as values, contacts with influential people, etc.

We also cannot ignore what these executives said about education as a preferred source of competence for certain activities. In Table 4 we have presented the activities in an array based on the scores for education only. While all the scores are low, it is instructive to examine their relative rankings. Two conclusions seem justified from the data. First, items with the highest scores, activities they think educators could help them with, are almost exclusively technical in nature. Second, items with low scores are role activities that are either inconsequential to the role or very crucial role activities requiring essentially political and human relations skills. Clearly, these executives see educators as technically oriented and ill-prepared to impart the skill these executives have already indicated in Table 3 that they see are best gained in the arena of life.

We used a second approach to gain information about educational preparation. Each respondent was asked to select five of the items in the standard list which he felt educators should stress in health service administration programs. (Table 5) There is a moderate correlation between the data in Tables 4 and 5–a correlation which should occur if respondents were consistent.

Perhaps the two most important conclusions which might be made from these data are: (1) although the health services administrator emphasizes the external environment, he generally does not see educators as able to provide him with much help in this area; and (2) although he feels interpersonal skills are best learned through experience or self-learning methods, he is wanting educators to stress influence processes. Considering the pluralistic structure within which the health service administrator must create bases of power, it is understandable why he would thus advocate the teaching of same. In a situation where one is first given responsibility and usually not granted sufficient authority and power to fulfill it properly, it is understandable that he would denigrate the normative-type management course he may have had in which it was taught that one was first given authority and subsequently expected to be held accountable for only those matters over which he was granted sufficient authority. While it may not be palatable for educators to be confronted with such data from practitioners, in cases where theory and practice diverge, it is theory that must yield to the reality it purports to represent. It would appear, therefore, that educators should consider these findings when making curriculum decisions.

TABLE 4

RELATIVE EMPHASIS ON EDUCATIONAL INSTITUTIONS AS
SOURCE OF COMPETENCE TO PERFORM ACTIVITIES

(Percentage of respondents who name some type of educational method as their first or second choice of gaining competence to perform executive activity. Question number given in parentheses at end of activity.)

%	Activity
39%	Decisions re: Quality control system procedures. (16)
37%	Employee/Management development, training. (24)
33%	Decisions re: Management information system. (30)
30%	Decisions re: Cost finding. (13)
30%	Decisions re: Organization structure. (29)
29%	Labor Negotiations. (14)
29%	Devising work procedures for nonprofessionals. (18)
28%	Decisions re: Medical-type records. (39)
27%	Decisions re: Diagnosis, i.e., Lab., EKG, X-ray, etc. (41)
26%	Devising work procedures for professionals. (17)
26%	Creating/changing professional jobs/units. (28)
26%	Long-range planning. (31)
25%	Decisions re: Treatment, i.e., medical, drugs, etc. (42)
24%	Market research. (1)
24%	Obtaining long-term capital. (10)
24%	Establishing agreements with other health organizations. (15)
23%	Public Relations. (3)
23%	Obtaining working capital; collections. (11)
23%	Arbitrate between policy-making groups (Boards, Staff, Administration). (45)
22%	Negotiating with powerful external organizations. (46)
21%	Determine buying procedures. (7)
21%	Scheduling, routing throughputs (patients). (19)
21%	Motivating immediate subordinates. (32)
20%	Influence decisions made by Board/Owners. (33)
20%	Decisions re: Dietary. (37)
19%	Decisions re: Nursing care. (36)
19%	Decisions re: Laundry and linen. (38)
19%	Decisions re: Housekeeping. (40)
18%	Lobbying and influencing government agency rulings. (4)
18%	Influence decisions made by the medical staff. (34)
14%	Project research. (2)
13%	Recruiting professionals, physicians. (22)
13%	Decisions re: new construction. (26)
12%	Transporting, distributing throughputs (patients). (6)
12%	Decisions re: maintaining building and equipment. (27)
12%	Dealing with personal and interpersonal problems. (43)
11%	Decisions re: appointments of physicians. (20)
11%	Routine work assignment scheduling. (23)
10%	Decisions re: professional and managerial salaries. (9)
10%	Rewarding professional and managerial employees. (21)
10%	Arbitrate between internal units, divisions. (44)
9%	Decisions re: charges/prices for services and products. (5)
8%	Disciplining professional/managerial employees. (25)
8%	Disciplining physicians. (35)
6%	New equipment decisions. (8)
2%	Approving exceptions to the budget of less than $500. (12)

TABLE 5
Items Educators Should Stress

Activity Number	Item	(f)
31(a)	Long-range planning for the organization	15
32(a)	Motivating and directing immediate subordinates	14
24(b)	Systematic development of employees i.e., mgt. development, empl. training.	13
3(c)	Influence public knowledge, opinion, or attitude.	12
30(a)	Decisions concerning financial and managerial type information.	12
16(d)	Developing criteria and systems to control quality of patient services.	11
33(e)	Influencing decisions made by Board/Owners.	9
43(a)	Dealing with personal and interpersonal problems.	8
45	Arbitrating, negotiating differences between medical staff, Board or owner, and administration.	6
29	Decide on changes in the authority structure, i.e., who reports to whom, committee membership, who is involved in decisions, etc.	5
34	Influencing decisions made by the Medical Staff.	5
14	Represent the organization in labor negotiations or disputes.	5
44	Arbitrating, negotiating differences between departments/units within organization.	4
46	Arbitrating, negotiating differences between us and influential coalitions and organizations outside our organization.	4
10	Obtaining long-term capital financing (stocks, bonds, loans, appropriations).	3
18	Devising or approving work procedures used by professionals.	3
22	Recruiting professional employees, physicians.	3

Notes:
(a) Mentioned by respondents from all four types of organizations.
(b) Mentioned chiefly by long-term care and clinics.
(c) Mentioned equally by all types of organizations except clinics. This is possibly clear difference between type i.e., the "market" for clinic manager is his captive M.D. panel, not "public" per se.
(d) Mentioned by only hospitals and long-term care—the two types most dependent on external financing from payors who can constrain!
(e) Mentioned by only hospitals and clinics.

We began our paper with a discussion of our theoretical perspective. The purpose was to indicate the issues we were sensitive to in our investigation rather than to set the stage for testing the theory or certain hypotheses. In retrospect, it appears the theory was both useful in developing a methodology for studying roles and in identifying key aspects of managerial function. Clearly, differences and commonalities among the four roles can be isolated and explained on the basis of the variables presented within the theory. Only a study involving larger numbers and random sampling techniques would permit definitive judgments about either the theory or the data. However, at the risk of being accused of seeing what we sought to see, it does appear that the open systems approach to organization structure and the decision theory or political models of decision making are closer approximations of reality than competing perspectives. In addition, it is clear these executives needed interpersonal and group process skills of the human relations type. It was less clear they needed to learn descriptive details of technical matters occurring in the production subsystems of their organizations. Generally speaking, they opt for either relying on experts or learning these details by experience.

Finally, this study raises even broader questions of knowledge versus values and training versus placement. Although we had no systematic method of collecting and analyzing our observations of such matters, we did become sensitized to the issue of certain personal characteristics and values that may be as important to success as the possession of discrete skills and knowledge. For example, it appears that to be hired and to remain as a medical group manager, one must hold values supportive to entrepreneurial medicine. Hence, one would be better advised to come to clinic management from the business school than through the public health school. Likewise, the consumer advocate might have problems in a foundation-type HMO but be quite at home in a prepaid group practice, consumer-oriented HMO such as the Group Health Cooperative of Puget Sound.

If values are as important as knowledge and skills, and self-instruction is a better source of competence than preparation in an educational institution, it follows logically that placement may be as important or more so than training. While we don't advocate such, we do feel it worthwhile for educators to be aware of these data and give these matters due consideration. For example, should values be a selection criterion in HSA programs and/or an explicit part of the curriculum? Should HSA programs reconsider their role in placement? Should HSA programs re-think the relative importance of on-campus and continuing education? Considering the priority practitioners place on "live action," current information as contrasted to dated/written information, should HSA programs re-think the definition of their product i.e., "education." If education is to become increasingly the on-line type knowledge of the external and internal organizational environments, then educators may well need to expand their domains into collecting and disseminating such information.

We don't maintain that our study offers data to answer such fundamental questions. It is sufficient that the study has raised what may be the right questions.

Notes

1. Warren G. Bennis. "Leadership Theory and Administrative Behavior: The Problem of Authority." *Administrative Science Quarterly*, December 1959. Vol. 4. pp. 259–301.
2. Ralph T. Murray, Paul R. Donnelly, and Margaret Threadgould. "How Administrators Spend Their Time." *Hospital Progress*, September 1968. pp. 49–58.
   Edward J. Connors and Joseph C. Hutts. "How Administrators Spend Their Day." *Hospitals*, February 1967. Vol. 41. pp. 45–50, 141.
   Donald E. Saathoff and Richard A. Kurtz. "What Administrators of Small Hospitals Do." *Modern Hospital*, August 1962. Vol. 99, No. 2. pp. 85–87, 142–147.
3. Paul R. Lawrence and Jay W. Lorsch. *Organization and Environment: Managing Differentiation and Integration*. Homewood, Illinois: Richard D. Irwin, Inc., 1969.
   Charles Perrow. "A Framework for the Comparative Analysis of Organizations." *American Sociological Review*, April 1967. Vol. 32, No. 2. pp. 194–208.
   Fred E. Fiedler. "A Contingency Model of Leadership Effectiveness." In L. Berkowitz, ed. *Advances in Experimental Social Psychology*. Vol. 1. pp. 149–190.
   D. S. Pugh, D. J. Hickson, C. R. Hinings, K. M. Macdonald, C. Turner, and T. Lupton. "A Conceptual Scheme for Organizational Analysis." *Administrative Science Quarterly*, December 1963. Vol. 8, No. 3. pp. 289–315.
4. Chester I. Barnard. *The Functions of the Executive*. Cambridge: Harvard University Press, 1938.
   Herbert A. Simon. *Administrative Behavior*, 2nd ed. New York: The Free Press, 1957.
   Richard M. Cyert and James G. March. *A Behavioral Theory of the Firm*. Englewood Cliffs, NJ: Prentice-Hall, Inc., 1963.
   Jeffery Pfeffer and Gerald R. Salancik. "Organizational Decision Making as a Political Process: The Case of a University Budget." *Administrative Science Quarterly*, June 1974. Vol. 19, No. 2, pp. 135–151.
5. Sol Levine and Paul E. White. "Exchange as a Conceptual Framework for the Study of Interorganizational Relationships." *Administrative Science Quarterly*, March 1969. Vol. 5. pp. 583–601.
   James D. Thompson and Frederick L. Bates. "Technology, Organization, and Administration." *Administrative Science Quarterly*, December 1957. Vol. 2, No. 3. pp. 325–343.
   David Jacobs. "Dependency and Vulnerability: An Exchange Approach to the Control of Organizations." *Administrative Science Quarterly*, March 1974. Vol., 19, No. 1. pp. 45–59.
6. Robert B. Duncan. "Characteristics of Organizational Environment and Perceived Environmental Uncertainty." *Administrative Science Quarterly*, September 1972. Vol. 17, No. 3. pp. 313–327.
7. Karl E. Weick. *The Social Psychology of Organizing*. Reading, MA: Addison-Wesley Pub. Co., 1969. pp. 63–71.

8. Daniel Katz and Robert L. Kahn. *The Social Psychology of Organizations.* New York: John Wiley and Sons, Inc., 1966.
9. Alan D. Bauerschmidt. "The Calculus of Hospital Administration." *Hospital Administration*, Fall 1971. Vol. 16. pp. 50–68.
   Richard T. Viguers. "The Politics of Power in a Hospital." *The Modern Hospital*, May 1961. Vol. 96, No. 5. pp. 89–94.
10. Howard E. Aldrich. "Technology and Organizational Structure: A Reexamination of the Findings of the Aston Group." *Administrative Science Quarterly*, March 1972. Vol. 17, No. 1. pp. 26–43.
    Wolf V. Heydebrand. *Hospital Bureaucracy: A Comparative Study of Organizations.* New York: Dunellen, 1973.
11. Charles Perrow. *Organizational Analysis: A Sociological View.* Belmont, CA: Wadsworth Pub. Co., Inc., 1970.
12. Ibid.
13. Miriam M. Johnson and Harry W. Martin. "A Sociological Analysis of the Nurse Role." In James K. Skipper, Jr. and Robert C. Leonard (eds.). *Social Interaction and Patient Care.* Philadelphia: J.B. Lippincott Co., 1965. pp. 29–39.
14. Wilbert Ellis Moore. *Order and Change: Essays in Comparative Sociology.* New York: John Wiley & Sons, Inc., 1967. pp. 175–180.
15. D. S. Pugh, D. J. Hickson, C. R. Hinings, and C. Turner. "Dimensions of Organization Structure." *Administrative Science Quarterly*, June 1968. Vol. 13. pp. 65–105.
16. Richard H. Hall. "The Concept of Bureaucracy: An Empirical Assessment." *American Journal of Sociology*, July 1963. Vol. 69, No. 1. pp. 32–40.
17. John Child. "Organization Structure and Strategies of Control: A Replication of the Aston Study." *Administrative Science Quarterly*, June 1972. Vol. 17, No. 2. pp. 163–177.
18. James G. March and Herbert A. Simon. *Organizations.* New York: John Wiley and Sons, Inc., 1958. p. 160.
19. David Mechanic. "Sources of Power of Lower Participants in Complex Organizations." *Administrative Science Quarterly*, December 1962. Vol. 7, No. 3. pp. 349–364.
20. James A. Knight, M.D. *Medical Student: Doctor in the Making.* New York: Appleton-Century Crofts, 1973. pp. 97–98.
21. Pugh et al. Ibid. Personal correspondence from Professor Pugh, June 19, 1973 in which he agrees that their first factor is similar to coordination by plans and procedures, Factor II is similar to hierarchical control by managers, and Factor III similar to self-peer control.
22. Jerald Hage and Michael Aiken. "Routine Technology, Social Structure, and Organizational Relationship." *Administrative Science Quarterly*, December 1969. Vol. 14, No. 3. pp. 366–376.
23. Richard H. Hall. "Some Organizational Considerations in the Profession-Organizational Relationship." *Administrative Science Quarterly*, December 1962. Vol. 7, No. 3. pp. 461–478.
24. Paul D. Montagna. "Professionalization and Bureaucratization in Large Professional Organizations." In Wolf V. Heydebrand. *Comparative Organ-*

izations: *The Results of Empirical Research.* Englewood Cliffs, NJ: Prentice-Hall, Inc., 1973. pp. 534–542.
25. Thompson and Bates. Ibid.
26. David J. Hickson, D. S. Pugh, and Diana C. Pheysey. "Operations Technology and Organization Structure: An Empirical Reappraisal." *Administrative Science Quarterly,* September 1969. Vol. 14, No. 3. pp. 378–397.
27. Allen Newell, J. C. Shaw, and Herbert A. Simon. "Elements of a Theory of Human Problem Solving." *Psychology Review,* 1958. Vol. 65, No. 3. pp. 151–166.
28. Harold H. Kelley and John W. Thibaut. "Group Problem Solving." In Gardner Lindzey and Elliot Aranson (eds.).*Handbook of Social Psychology.* Reading, MA: Addison-Wesley Pub. Co. pp. 69–70.
29. Perrow. Op. cit.
30. Pugh (1968). Op. cit. Child. Op. cit.
31. Pugh (1968). Op. cit.
32. George Strauss and Leonard R. Sayles. *Personnel: The Human Problems of Management,* 3rd ed. Englewood Cliffs, NJ: Prentice-Hall, Inc., 1972. p. 324.
33. Aldrich. Op. cit.
34. Katz and Kahn. Op. cit.
35. Pugh (1968). Op. cit.
36. Joseph L. Fleiss. "Measuring Nominal Scale Agreement Among Many Raters." *Psychology Bulletin.* Vol. 76, No. 5. pp. 378–382.
37. Richard J. Light. "Measures of Response Agreement for Qualitative Data: Some Generalizations and Alternatives." *Psychology Bulletin.* Vol. 76, No. 5. pp. 365–377.
38. Henry Mintzberg. *The Nature of Managerial Work.* New York: Harper & Row, 1973.
39. Harold Koontz and Cyril O'Donnell. *Principles of Management: An Analysis of Managerial Functions.* New York: McGraw-Hill Book Co., Inc., 1955. pp. 22–28.
40. John R. Campbell, M. Dunnette, Ed Lawler, and Karl Weick. *Managerial Behavior, Performance, and Effectiveness.* New York: McGraw-Hill, 1970. pp. 74–81.
41. *Nursing Home Fact Book 1970–1.* Washington, D.C.: The American Nursing Home Association. p. 72.
42. John V. Therrell. "Top Management — In the Middle." *Medical Group Management,* July 1972. Vol. 19, No. 5. pp. 6–8.
43. Dorwin Cartwright. "Influence, Leadership, and Control." In James G. March (ed). *Handbook of Organizations.* Chicago: Rand McNally & Co., 1965. pp. 1–47.
44. Tom Burns and G. M. Stalker. *The Management of Innovation.* London: Tavistock Publications, 1961. p. 123.
    Bertram M. Gross. *The Managing of Organizations.* New York: The Free Press, 1964. p. 497.
45. C. J. Haberstroh. "Organization Design and Systems Analysis." In James G. March (ed.). *Handbook of Organizations.* Chicago: Rand McNally & Co., 1965. p. 1184.

46. Kenneth R. Andrews. "Toward Professionalism in Business Management." *Harvard Business Review*, March–April 1969. Vol. 47, No. 2, pp. 49–60.
47. C. Wright Mills. "The Chief Executives." In Barney G. Glaser (ed.). *Organizational Careers: A Sourcebook for Theory*. Chicago: Aldine Pub. Co., 1968. pp. 417–425.
48. Renato Tagiuri. "Value Orientations and the Relationship of Managers and Scientists." *Administrative Science Quarterly*, June 1965. Vol. 10, No. 1. pp. 39–51.
    Burns and Stalker. Op. cit. pp. 104–119.
    Robert Presthus. *The Organizational Society*. New York: Alfred A. Knopf, Inc., 1962. p. 438.
49. T. R. Sarbin and Vernon L. Allen. "Role Theory." In Gardner Lindzey and Eliot Aranson (eds.). *The Handbook of Social Psychology*, 2nd ed. Vol. 1. Reading, MA: Addison-Wesley Pub. Co., 1968. p. 555.

Part IV

Papers Presented at the
Institute on New
Approaches to Education for
Health Administration

Authors in Part IV

James R. Kimmey, M.D., M.P.H.
Secretary of Health
Policy Council of the State of Wisconsin

George A. Lamb, M.D.
Associate Professor
Department of Preventive and Social Medicine
Harvard Medical School

Jerry W. Miller, Ph.D.
Director, Office on Educational Credit
American Council on Education

Fred E. Mondragon, M.B.A.
Administrator, Bernalillo County Medical Center
Albuquerque, New Mexico

Stephen B. Plumer, Ph.D.
Education Consultant
Potomac, Maryland

William C. Richardson, Ph.D.
Associate Professor and Chairman
 Department of Health Services
School of Public Health and Community Medicine
University of Washington

Julius B. Richmond, M.D.
Professor and Chairman
 Department of Preventive and Social Medicine
Hairvard Medical School

Nathan J. Stark
Vice Chancellor for Health Affairs
University of Pittsburgh

David B. Starkweather, Dr. P.H.
Director
Graduate Curriculum in Hospital Administration
School of Public Health
University of California, Berkeley

Public Accountability and Human Services Orientation in Health Administration*

Introduction

The American health care non-system, and the educational community which prepares its administrators, must undergo a complete re-orientation. There must be correlation and communication between the health care hierarchy (students, educators, and practitioners) and the community (individual patients, government, third party payers, employees, society). The needs and values of society must be reflected in the practices and values of those who would serve that society.

The above-sounded theme, and a proposed model for educators and practitioners in the health administration arena, are developed in this paper. The paper attempts to deal with the issues of public accountability and human services orientation in health administration. The model suggests a re-orientation for educators, students and practitioners, away from the organizational and educational process and setting, and toward the people served: the public and the individual patient.

The guidelines to authors suggested that authors develop a new approach to education for health administration that would be innovative and reflect an advocacy position. Since original thought is usually a distillation of education, experience and readings, it would be arrogant to claim originality in this attempt.

The structure of the discussion shall involve a short statement of forces working counter to accountability and human orientation, a discussion of several specific issues, and a development of the model to improve performance in these areas.

* by Fred E. Mondragon

The Problem

There are forces, internal and external to health care organizations, which contribute to deficiencies in public accountability and human services orientation in health care organizations. These may be divided into the two categories, although there may be overlapping, particularly in regard to the lack of feedback mechanisms.

Forces Adversely Affecting Human Services Orientation

The forces which create deficiencies in human services orientation in health care situations include the size and complexity of health care organizations and the effects of the new professions. Size affects this orientation due to the problems of organizational distance between the people who determine the objectives of the organization and the employees who deliver the actual care. The objective of personal, kind, high quality care, often becomes diluted in its transmission down the organizational ladder and is sometimes supplanted by individual goals of the deliverer of care or by loyalty to a procedure or system. Conversely, organizational distance may deprive the administrator of valuable "front line" feedback from patients and employees regarding goals and procedures for delivering high quality individualized care.

Organizational and environmental complexity is an important factor in detracting from human services orientation. A health administrator must deal with such issues as new federal regulations for capital expenditures, third party regulations, Phase IV guidelines, a tenuous financial position, labor contracts, architectural discussions and legal issues. The technical aspects of hospital administration require a time commitment of such magnitude that the administration slights the important human services aspects of hospital operation.

A third factor which hurts the patient orientation is loyalty to individual professions as opposed to patient care considerations. The ultraprofessionals, both in the medical and business segments of the hospital, sometimes tend to ignore the human needs of the patient in favor of procedural matters or professional, sometimes arbitrary, barriers. The unresponsiveness and arrogance of the health professionals prevent the feedback necessary to inform the administrator and the hospital staff of deficiencies in the system. This is particularly true when the individual receiving the service is stripped of his clothes, his dignity and is made to feel depersonalized in the strange world of the hospital.

Forces Adversely Affecting Public Accountability

There are several factors contributing to the lack of public accountability in the health care system. The first is a deficiency in the educational system for hospital administration. The technical and administrative courses require such great effort that there is no space in curriculum for courses in practical politics and no time for involvement by the student in community relationships.

Secondly, the structure of community hospital governance is such that the administrator is responsible, for all practical purposes, to no one. Community hospital boards are neither representative of the community nor an effective counter-force to hospital management. The Committee for Economic Development phrased the problem succinctly in the publication, *Building a National Health Care System:*

> The member who spends one luncheon a month with the hospital board cannot possibly learn enough about the workings of the hospital to do anything more than rubber-stamp the administrator and the medical staff.[1]

Thus the community hospital system becomes a system of baronies fitting the description by Anthony Jay in his book, *Management and Machiavelli:*

> ... the basic political unit of Anglo-Norman times was the feudal overlord with his manor, his surrounding land and their revenues, and his more or less dependent peasantry ... To be an English baron in the twelfth century ... was to exercise independent, arbitary, and unfettered power ...[2]

The public hospitals, although forced by their mission to interact with political forces in the community through elected officials, often became the victims of the politicians, to be plundered for political purposes. The oligarchy changes from self-appointed to selfish-elected. The administrator is either an insulated driver or a harassed administrative technician, with the community, in either case, exercising no significant influence over hospital policies.

Another significant force working counter to public accountability in health administration is the pressure of internal accountabilities. The problems of balanced budgets, cash flow, proper organization and planning, employee demands and complex regulations are overwhelming. They demand attention to the point that the health administrator cannot deal with external accountabilities. Internal concerns and problems can sometimes overtake an administrator and literally bankrupt the organization if proper business acumen is not exercised and if the administrator devotes too much valuable time to external concerns. The administrator must be assured that internal problems are stable if public accountability is to be dealt with properly.

The Issues

In order to understand the educational requirements to make the administrator sensitive to the needs of the individual patients and the public, it is necessary to explore in greater detail the principles of human services orientation and public accountability. Several issues are discussed as they relate to the two principles under discussion.

HIGH QUALITY, HIGHLY INDIVIDUALIZED SERVICES IN A LARGE-SCALE ORGANIZATION

Nothing infuriates a sensitive administrator more than to witness a cold impersonal response to a patient by a nurse, a discussion by professionals about a patient's disease in the patient's presence, as if the patient were not there, or the reference to a patient by disease, as in "the hernia in 438." If the administrator is sensitive, how can that sensitivity be transferred to the employees, who have the greatest contact with the patient and the public? This is one of the most frustrating problems for administrators, since, regardless of the number of times the organizational goals of patient care are repeated, the tyranny of procedures and the arrogance of professionalism are sometimes insurmountable.

In order to assure compliance, the administrator may utilize the traditional organizational principles of planning, organizing, and control to assure compliance with organizational goals. These principles, particularly the control principle, apply negative sanctions to violators of rules which may be promulgated regarding the treatment of patients and high quality procedures.

However, sanctions by themselves do not result in the highly humanized care, manifested by the extra kindness most appreciated by patients. More importantly, the employee must be inspired to provide the friendly personalized care which the employee would expect if the roles of patient and employee reversed. The inspiration for the employee must come, directly or indirectly, from the chief executive of the hospital. The administrator's relationships with subordinates are reflected in relations with subsequent organizational levels, and finally in the employee's one-to-one interaction with the patient.

The administrator's sense of values and human worth will be discussed later in the paper; however, at this point it would be useful to discuss several organizational techniques which can assist the administrator to assure that high quality personal care is provided and to provide valuable feedback from patients and employees.

The patient advocate. Although some administrators may claim that *all* employees are patient advocates, they are usually sadly mistaken. The sensitive administrator should appoint a patient advocate or "ombudsperson" to assist patients in dealing with the hospital hierarchy. This is particularly important in public hospitals where minority or poor patients may not understand the language, the system, and the rights of patients.

The open door. Some secretaries and assistants hold the belief that the administrator's office is a sanctuary that can be violated only at the express request of the lord of the manor. The tendency of immediate subordinates to protect is probably a reflection of the administrator's desires. It is easy to declare "open door" policy, but many an administrator subsequently tolerates the harassment by assistants and secretaries of patients who may wish to call or speak to the administrator personally. The practice of receiving spontaneous visitors lends more credibility to an open-door policy than the protestations of a memorandum.

Freedom to circulate. Despite the operational pressures upon the administrator it is important that enough time be set aside to circulate throughout the hospital to observe directly the activities and actions of individuals in the organization. This circulation inspires pride in the employees that the administrator takes an interest in their work. Another valuable function of visiting different areas of the hospital is to provide feedback from patients and employees. Many deficiencies and improvements may be discovered by the administrator through direct contact with patients and employees.

Management by objectives. In its most elementary form, the principle of management by objectives provides a common thread through which employees can identify with the goals of the hospital. Hospital management can utilize a number of vehicles to distribute and reinforce the objective of high quality, personal care to patients. One important means of reinforcing the patient care objectives of the organization is for the administrator to make the individual patient and his care a constant point of reference in all administrative decisions and plans. The articulation of this orientation as frequently as possible will inspire others in the organization to retain their human services orientation.

Participatory Democracy in Administration — The New Realities

Much has been written about the principle of participation in decision making. Sharing decision making with subordinates has the obvious advantages of allowing the persons charged with implementing policy to develop it, thereby causing the subordinate to share ownership in the policy and responsibility for its implementation. It now appears that participatory democracy is becoming a non-optional reality in many organizations. For example, labor unions have become an effective counter-force, influencing labor and economic policy as well as quality of care policy, as in the case of the House Staff Union lawsuit against a California County Hospital to force certain improvements. Legal recourse is another means of forced participation in decision making. A lawsuit, or the threat of a suit may influence the administrator's deliberations and decision.

New management arrangements, such as matrix organization are forcing administrators to consult with team leaders and functional directors. In addition, theoretically there is enough lateral coordination that the administrator may not need to be involved in some decisions at all. As stated by Neuhauser, "The concept of the matrix organization brings into focus the importance of the patient care team for lateral coordination and the need for promoting team management."[3]

There are other means by which the administrator can be forced to engage in participatory democracy. Militant groups, pursuing a particular course, may bring an entire organization to a halt by strategically planned interruptions as described by Alvin Toffler; ". . . in the new, fast-paced cybernetic society a minority can, by sabotage, strike, or a thousand other means, disrupt the entire system."[4]

Public Accountability — The New Rules

Public accountability of health care institutions has not been attempted in governmental policy in this country prior to 1965. The Hill-Burton program, notwithstanding its requirement for a state hospital plan did little to contribute to health planning. Although many excellent institutions were established and expanded with the assistance of Hill-Burton grants, in many cases senseless overbedding and self-serving empire building occurred.

The Medicare-Medicaid law, passed in 1965, included, for the first time, national criteria for hospital reimbursement. The application of these criteria, plus the legitimatization of the utilization review process, presented a first step by the Federal Government toward accountability for actions by individual hospitals. Hospitals could no longer engage in totally arbitrary charge setting, since retroactive cost settlements forced a relationship between costs and charges. There were no constraints, however, over costs and capital expenditures. The years following the implementation of the Medicare law represented years of rampant inflation in health care costs and charges.

Public Law 92-603 was another significant step in forcing hospital public accountability in the areas of quality review and capital expenditures. Section 1122 now requires review of Comprehensive Health Planning Agencies and Designated Planning Agencies for capital expenditures costing more than $100,000, and for the initiation of a new service. The professional standards review organization section promises to exert a significant influence over medical care in the hospital.

The uncoordinated attempts by the Federal Government to force public accountability in hospital operation were expanded by the Economic Stabilization program in 1972 and 1973. Phases I through IV are further regulatory mechanisms through which financial restraint and responsibility have been incorporated in public policy.

Other efforts to bring about public accountability in hospitals include the new public disclosure law in California, certificate of need legislation in several states and rate setting laws. In addition, the public hearing requirement of the Joint Commission on Accreditation of Hospitals also attempts to solicit public feedback regarding hospital services.

Federal regulations, state legal requirements, and voluntary accrediting agency controls represent attempts to make health administrators more accountable to the public. Public accountability, however, demands that the administrator become involved in a continual dialogue with the hospital's community. The dialogue may take place in the organizational context or in the political arena.

Policy-maker and Politician — The New Roles

The complexities of hospital operation make the administrator much more than a caretaker and coordinator in the hospital organization. Difficult policy decisions must be recommended to boards of trustees and medical staff organizations by the administrator. This leadership in the health care field requires as a prerequisite that the administrator become the master of the internal organization, since the administrator would lose credibility in attempting to be a change agent if the organization is faltering.

Having conquered the complexities of hospital management, the administrator can engage in statesmanship both within and without the health care system. Many administrators become the prime architects of hospital progress, devoting time to educate physicians and trustees properly and to becoming agents for change which will benefit the public and the patients.

The administrator should participate in community activities, to serve the community with the vast amounts of organizational ability usually possessed by managers of complex institutions. This community contact not only lends more opportunity for the administrator to influence community decisions but also provides valuable feedback to the administrator regarding needs, values and demands. The administrator cannot afford to work in a vacuum; and community contact provides more direct information, unsolicited and unscreened by boards or internal barriers.

The militant stance taken collectively by health administrators recently in the response to Phase IV regulations indicated a further role of the administrator as a change agent vis-a-vis the Federal Government. Hospital administrators have little right to complain about arbitrary regulations or discriminatory guidelines if they do not attempt, to the maximum limits possible, to influence the setting of such regulations. This may include direct political involvement, either legitimized, as in the regional councils of health in some Canadian provinces or informal activity, as in the domestic political process. In regard to the latter process, the administrator must be wary lest the relationship with regulatory agencies and political contacts become a new corrupt symbiosis, as the Watergate horror stories have warned us.

Politics has recently obtained an unpleasant connotation: at their best, the art and practice of politics provide an opportunity for the health administrator to act as change agent and, additionally, to learn the needs and values of the community and become more accountable. Richard H. Seder writing in the *American Journal of Public Health* describes the political process:

> Politics will be used to mean the identification of popular concerns, the assessment of value and power distribution in a population and its subparts, the evaluation of the public and special interest groups, and the negotiation of acceptable courses of action and resource use—almost always compromises—across the set of interested parties.[5]

Politics as a change-process is valuable for a health administrator. However, the person who attempts change must be assured that the change represents a positive contribution to health care and society as reflected in community needs and values. Ethics and values of the community should be interpreted by the health administrator in the context of the administrator's own values. The next section deals with human values in the administrator.

ETHICS IN HEALTH ADMINISTRATION

The matter of ethics and values is paramount in discussing the health administrator's stance toward public accountability and human services orientation. As we have read in recent newspaper accounts, executives are not exempt from the temptations of buying favors, of kickbacks, extortion, spying and sabotage. The apparent erosion of ethics is a symptom of moral decay and erosion of values and ethics in our public and private sectors. The health administrator must constantly wrestle with questions of ethics and values.

Any doubts about the existence of ethical considerations are erased by examining some current issues and their subjection to value judgments. The matter of determining cerebral death, the question of abortion, the granting of surgical privileges to an incompetent surgeon, the ethics of certain types of medical research, and the duplication of unnecessary facilities for self-aggrandizement are all matters which involve the health administrator's value system. The feelings toward minority individuals may reflect a health administrator's values and ethics produced in early development. (Would the syphilis experimentation among blacks in the South and the deceptive contraceptive research among Mexican-American women in Texas have occurred if the subjects had not been minority persons? Was there not a health administrator in the health research establishment or in the Federal funding structure who could have had the moral strength to intercept the process?)

The sensitivity and feelings of a health administrator toward the public and the individual patient will influence every decision and plan made in the organizational context. The manager's attitudes and beliefs will be mirrored in the values and attitudes of the organization and its individual members. The book *Managers for Tomorrow* phrased the concept in the following way: "An organization is the structural aspect of a philosophy, while administration is the implementation of that philosophy."[6]

Values assist in singling out what is and is not important. Many a decision made by a health administrator is made by considering whether the choice is for the ultimate benefit of the patient and/or community served by the hospital. A positive attitude on the part of the administrator toward the people served provides a feeling of security, a protection from panic in the face of crises, and a solid base for the health administrator to plan and execute without succumbing to confusion, harassment, intemperate action, or gimmickery.

However, according to Flory, "Few people possess a well-articulated system of values. Yet most of what one does is directed by basic attitudes toward self and others, by certain ideas of success, by concepts of personal responsibility, and by meaning attached to life itself. Everyone continually makes value judgements."[7] How does an administrator develop feelings toward his communities after his values are determined? Can values be altered in the educational process and in the administrator's working situation? In the practitioner's world, it is important that the health administrator organize available time sufficiently well so that there is ample opportunity for reflection, community interchange and individual patient contact. The inculcation of community values and needs into the administrator's thinking must then be further developed and nurtured in the organizational philosophy and values.

In the educational setting, ethics and values must be developed, not by imposing the educator's values but, in the words of Alvin Toffler, educators must "systematically organize formal and informal activities that help the student define, explicate and test his values, whatever they are. Our schools will continue to turn out industrial men until we teach young people the skills necessary to identify and clarify, if not reconcile, conflicts in their own value systems."[8] In this context, it is critical that educational institutions, including health care administration schools, expand their curricula to include opportunities for meaningful exchange with communities, local and regional. This community interchange, as practiced by the U.S.C. and Cincinnati programs, is a positive force in making the schools more responsive and in teaching sensitivity and accountability to health administration students.

The Model

The model for health administration practice and education for the future must, of necessity, revolve around the community. This is particularly true if the student, the educator, and the health administration practitioner are to develop public accountability and human services orientation. The most obvious interactions in the model are those between student and teacher. The student presents challenges, the teacher imparts knowledge. Relations must also be developed between practitioner and educator and between student and practitioner. The advantages of such interchange are more obvious and will not be dwelt upon.

The uniqueness of the proposed model, if there is a grain of novelty, is the interaction between the student and the community, between the educator and the community and between the practitioner and the community. The student develops values and beliefs from interaction with the community in developmental years. The educator must constantly experience community contact and accountability in order

MODEL FOR HEALTH ADMINISTRATION EDUCATION AND PRACTICE

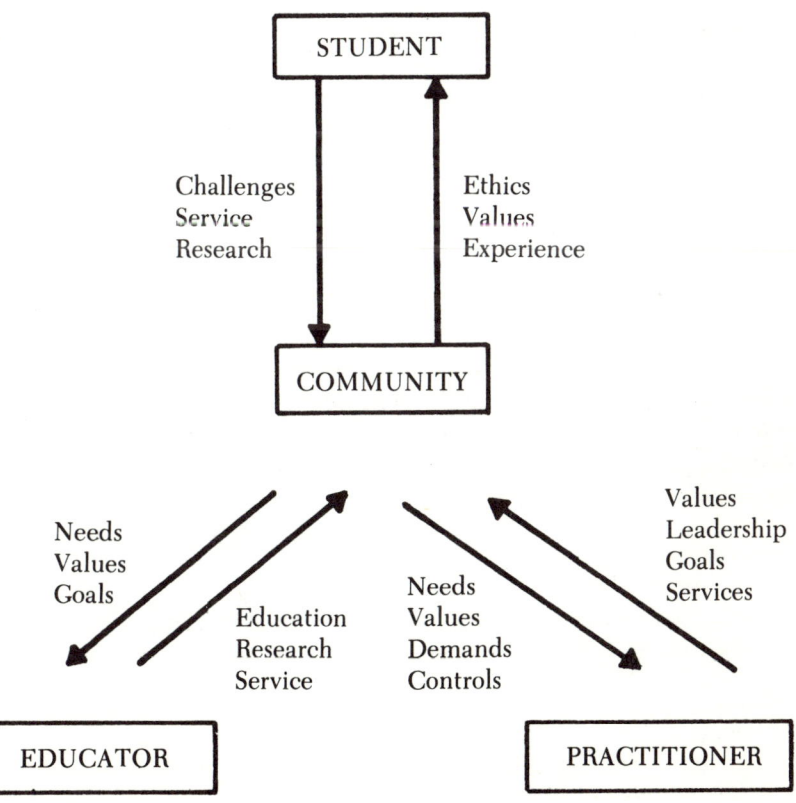

to teach accountability and human orientation. And the practicing health administrator must continually communicate with forces in the community and individual patients to maintain a proper orientation and *raison d'etre*. In the words of Dr. Michael Crichton, "The addition of community clinics, separate from the hospital, will almost certainly change the psychological set of doctors working within the physical setting of the hospital itself."[9] The same may be said for health administration students, educators and practitioners.

In this context the community may be defined as consumers (individual patients), consumer groups, politicians, poverty groups, institutions, government, employees, and others—in a word, society. The administrator, teacher, and student must continually engage in creative communication and mutual impartation of values and needs.

The concept of community-oriented schools in teaching health professionals has been proposed by Ellis: "Formal courses will become rare and be replaced by work-learn programs of community action problems. The students learn that which they need to know to solve problems in the community . . . Higher education will become essentially a community extension program."[10] Alvin Toffler also forecasts that students will be taught by adults in the community. Curriculum will be shaped by students and community groups.[11]

SUMMARY

This paper has attempted to discuss the issues of public accountability and human services orientation in health administration. A short description of the reasons for a decline in these orientations was followed by a discussion of several issues involved in the subject. Finally a new model for the practice and teaching of health administration was presented which emphasizes the role of the community in influencing and determining the values of health administration students, educators, and practitioners.

NOTES

1. Committee for Economic Development. *Building a National Health Care System.* New York: The Committee for Economic Development, 1973. p. 47.
2. Anthony Jay. *Management and Machiavelli.* New York: Holt Rinehart and Winston, 1968. p. 41.
3. Duncan Neuhauser. "The Hospital as a Matrix Organization." *Hospital Administration,* Fall 1972. pp. 8-25.

4. Alvin Toffler. *Future Shock.* New York: Random House, 1970. p. 477.
5. Richard H. Seder. "Planning and Politics and the Allocation of Health Resources." *American Journal of Public Health,* September 1973. Vol. 63, No. 9. p. 774.
6. Charles D. Flory. *Managers for Tomorrow.* New York: Mentor Books, 1967. pp. 23, 24.
7. Ibid. p. 215.
8. Toffler. Op. cit. pp. 417, 418.
9. Michael Crichton. *Five Patients: The Hospital Explained.* New York: Alfred A. Knopf, 1970. p. 205.
10. Edward V. Ellis. "A Human Development Approach to the Education and Training of New Health Professionals." Paper presented at the American Public Health Association Meeting, San Francisco, CA, November 8, 1973.
11. Toffler. Op. cit. pp. 406, 407.

Putting Health Into Health Administration*

Introduction

Many of the features of health administration in modern United States reflect the concerns of western medicine over the past several centuries. Historically, the English word "health" was apparently first used around 1000 A.D. to indicate a sense of soundness. At a somewhat later time the meaning also included a moral and spiritual soundness as well, with a definite religious significance.[1] In the more modern times, health has been defined in the context of a disease-free state or condition. Thus, "illness" administration may have been a more appropriate label than health administration. As noted by Brody the "traditional view" of medical practice and administration has "assumed the existence of a set of discrete entities called diseases and a set of other entities called therapies or therapeutic agents. These two sets were thought to be related in an imperfect 1:1 correspondence. The task of the physician was to classify signs and symptoms to determine which disease entities were present in his patient. When successful, this process of diagnosis suggested the corresponding therapy which the physician was to apply."[2] Health was considered to be only the absence of illness.

Disease has continued largely to be the emphasis of medicine, and thus of health administration to the present time. The tremendous impetus of the advances in pathology, microbiology and pharmacology of the nineteenth and twentieth centuries only emphasized and strengthened the disease model. The resulting research and therapeutic and preventive approaches founded in specific illness therapy have been thought by many to be the major factors in decreasing illness and death in the last few decades. Kass has suggested that although therapeutic approach to illness has had some effect on life expectancy, most

---

* by George A. Lamb and Julius B. Richmond.

of the decrease in morbidity, particularly that caused by infectious agents, has resulted instead from social change and public health measures.[3] Certainly as a consequence of the illness orientation, the health profession has measured illness and disease with terms such as morbidity and mortality, and rates of hospitalization, operation and specific illnesses (respiratory disease, myocardial infarction, etc.). Indeed, Stewart noted in 1970 that, "It is not possible to count health. However, it is possible to count death, disability, and disease in a population. Thus, an assessment of the health of Americans is arrived at . . ."[4] Only tangentially have we talked about health and this in such areas as life expectancy, productivity, and occasionally the quality of life.

Many of the presently effective preventive measures were developed in the last century to eradicate and ameliorate disease. These approaches have included primary (prevention of disease as with immunization), secondary (prevention of disease progression) and tertiary (rehabilitation of the ill).[5] The role of personal function (within society) as a component of health was noted by Pease and Crocker in 1943, in the Peckham Experiment. ". . . it became clear that while operating efficiently as a scene for the detection of disease and disorder, periodic health overhaul is ineffective as a health measure in the absence of 'instruments of health' providing conditions in and through which the biological potentiality of the family can find expression."[6]

The continuing focus on pathology and illness in this country by the health professions has also had its impact on the expectations of the American population without regard to the cultural aspects of health. In most of the concepts one must recognize that varying cultures may have different health goals. Lamm states, "The duty of the medical profession is to exert criticism on the 'health market,' to educate people toward a better recognition of the interaction between mode of life and development to disease, and to find more and more 'risk factors' of future ill health and elaborate ways for their elimination. Unfortunately, there is practically no market for these goals and nobody wants to pay the bill."[7] Thus, we continue to offer, and the public continues to buy, coronary artery bypass surgery, and heart transplantation, rather than diet control, exercise, elimination of smoking, etc. Only with difficulty have we persuaded some groups to seek care for the promotion of health (children, some professionals, military, unions). Even here these services are largely available only for those who can afford them and are used relatively ineffectively.

Health Taxonomy

In looking at health, we recognize the relative dearth of nomenclature, partly because of the heavy historical emphasis on disease and pathology. Indeed, the usual coding of medical diagnosis (ICDA) has been linked to the problems of hospitalized patients. Some adaptations have been necessary for ambulatory patients and even more changes will be necessary for those seeking health maintenance. In the founding of the World Health Organization, newer perspectives (or perhaps more ancient) were added when health was defined as ". . . a state of complete physical, mental, and social well being and not merely the absence of disease or infirmity."[8] This broad definition has proved to be difficult to use practically and thus there is still considerable need for health nomenclature.[9]

A multifactorial, dynamic conceptual view of optimal health was proposed by Richmond and Lustman in 1954.[10] Figure 1 presents a visual representation of optimal health (with an arbitrary inner circle area of 100) with emphasis on the interactions between this and the internal, external, and emotional environments. Figure 2 illustrates the usefulness of the visual aid in an asthmatic child where the indentations of the health circle depict a condition of suboptimal health and outpocketing is an adaptation toward health. This visual presentation allows one to understand that optimal health may be lacking even in the absence of symptoms. That this may occur very often was recognized by Pease and Crocker who found that 59 percent of their population appeared to be in a state of well-being, when, in fact, a disorder (or ill health) was present but not manifest.[11] In this context it is the task of the health care system to move people and society toward the spectrum of optimal health. In defining this goal in another way, Sigerist indicates that medicine is a social science, stating, "There can be no doubt that the target of medicine is to keep individuals adjusted to their environment as useful members of society, or readjust them when they have dropped out as a result of illness. It is a social goal . . ."[12]

Other approaches to the nomenclature of health have further emphasized the functional capacity of individuals. Fanshel defines health as, "A person is well if he is able to carry on his usual daily activities. To the extent that he cannot, he is in a state of dysfunction, or deviation from well-being."[13] In this context, he develops a scale of health (health status index) and demonstrates its usefulness with the example of venereal disease. It is a particularly helpful model in that it deals

FIGURE 1

HOMEOSTATIC CAPACITY OF ORGANISM*

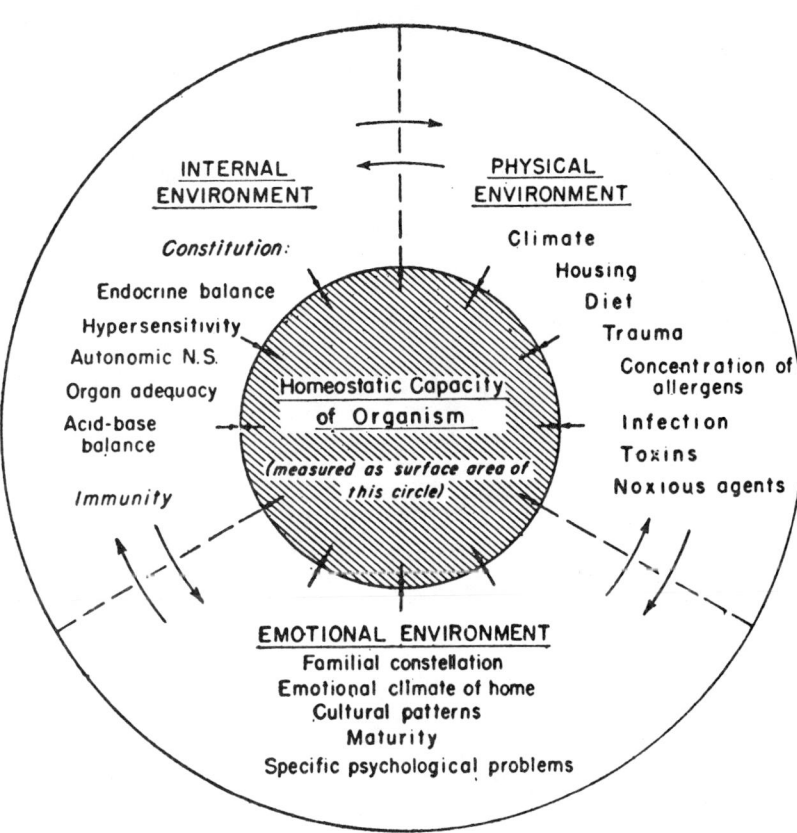

* Reproduced from *Journal of Medical Education*, January, 1954 with the permission of the publisher.

FIGURE 2

MULTIFACTIONAL IMPACT OF ASTHMA ON HEALTH*

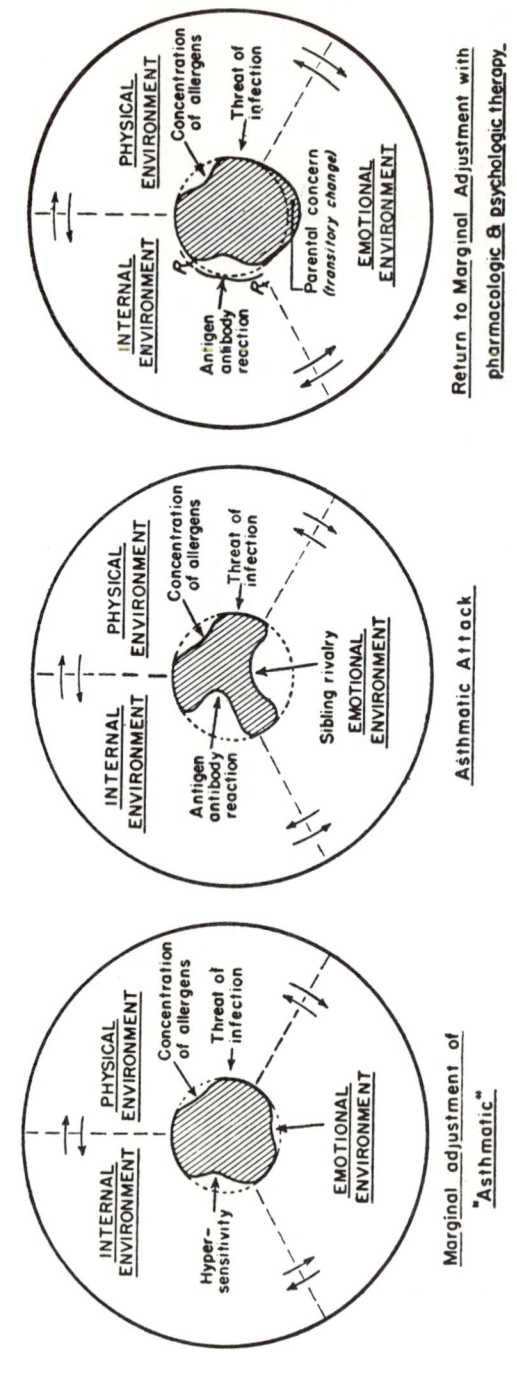

* Reproduced from *Journal of Medical Education*, January, 1954 with permission of the publisher.

with length of time that the dysfunction persists as well as the type of dysfunction. He also points out that the diagnostic and therapeutic approaches may themselves be dysfunctional and detract from optimal health.

Breslow carries the health index approach further in describing the work of the Human Population Laboratory of Almeda County, California.[14] He suggests that a person's perception of his (her) sense of well-being and that of an outside observer might be included in the health index as well as the function-dysfunction approach (performance of daily duties). Rosser and Watts demonstrated this with a theoretical model of a health index allowing a distinction between the observable state of function and the person's subjective state of well-being.[15] However, there is no clear way to weight the different perceptions of well-being when comparing the different ratings by self and other. These and other suggestions for a health index have tended to be very specific, mathematical and often quite detailed.[16-19] However, intricate equations and calculations indeed may not be necessary. Fanshel notes, "It is also helpful to point out that to quantify a concept does not require the high precision of some of the measurements found in the physical sciences. It may be, that for a more rational approach to the health services, it is sufficient to establish the order of magnitude."[20]

Many of these indices suggest that an entirely new scale which is continuous be developed in place of the dichotomous suggestions of illness and health so engrained in medicine.[21] The analogy of this approach to the measurement of heat and cold with a thermometer is obvious although the practical resolution is again less clear. Previous commonly used terms in this context include "the walking wounded," "weller-than-well," and "fit for light duty." The scales suggested by Richmond and Lustman,[22] Fanshel[23] and Breslow[24] describe a continuum of health to non-health in the thermometer context.

Finally, just as there is need for emphasis on and improvement in the terminology of health, there is also an urgency in developing the technology to apply health indices for use in outcome measures. The traditional measurements of health services have included change in morbidity and mortality rates (infant, maternal, age and disease specific, etc.), life expectancy, rates of hospitalization, rates of specific illnesses and so forth. In looking at the use of statistics, The Committee to Evaluate the National Center for Health Statistics has recommended the development of indices of health status and noted that "The primary role of health statistics in the United States should be: 1) to provide a comprehensive picture of the nature and magnitude of the nation's health problems; 2) to assess how well health services are meeting these problems, at what cost, and with what gain; and 3) to serve basic health research needs."[25] Thus, in addition to the usual cost-benefit financial type of analysis, other features of health need to be looked at to answer the question "with what gain."

Health in Health Administration

Arm in arm with medicine health administration has given a high priority to illness and little or none to health in the more modern sense. For example, the single largest expense in the United States health sphere in 1972 was hospital care, approximately 32.5 billion dollars (or 39 percent of the health dollar). Hospital care for the ill instead of ambulatory care or health promotion often has been emphasized because of political and economic forces. Many of the reimbursement mechanisms have promoted the expensive in-hospital care with little or no incentive for appropriate ambulatory care or health maintenance. Similarly, the financial need to maintain high bed occupancy in hospitals has undoubtedly led to higher hospitalization rates. Even in the prepaid plans where some financial incentives for ambulatory care are included, the basic cost of hospital beds is included, and increased group income is realized if the beds are kept full. To some extent hospital beds have been generated by medical technology without proven effectiveness of the technique or its concomitant hospitalization.[26] The tremendously rapid increase in the number and complexity of coronary care units is an example of providing expensive, in-hospital services of essentially unproven benefit.[27] Furthermore, many of the services, (involving monitors, noise, impersonality, limited visiting, etc.) may only serve to augment the anxiety of the patient and detract from the quality of health as well. Thus, we need to reconsider the proper environment for many of the ill and recognize that the relatively sterile, noisy hospital may further decrease health.[28] The importance of family participation in patient care[29] and in the vital decisions regarding the care for their loved ones cannot be overemphasized. Certainly, some health services may need to be provided at home or in an ambulatory setting rather than in the hospital even though this may be inconvenient for the provider and generate less payment (at least under present mechanisms). Within the hospital, accommodations must be made for the family: liberalizing visiting hours, teaching and allowing the family to deliver health services, and involving them in life and death decisions.[30-32]

Health administration could provide a new impetus in these directions. Financial or other incentives to decrease bed occupancy within hospitals, payment by illness (e.g., appendectomy) rather than on a per diem basis, and hospital education programs (e.g., accident prevention) might well be examples. In addition, there will need to be further public, financial, and professional acceptance of the importance of health promotion. Perhaps here we may get back to some of the ancient Chinese concepts of payment as it applies to our country. Thus, if a child develops measles (rubeola), an eminently preventable disease, because of the lack of provision of immunization,[33] the cost of the illness should not be the family's responsibility. Indeed, perhaps "the inferior doctor" in this case should assume at least the financial burden. This says nothing of the emotional, developmental and intellectual costs of the disease to the patient and his family. A similar analysis is now indicated in comparing the costs of diet control (cholesterol and caloric) and anti-hypertensive therapy in the control of coronary-artery disease to the cost of coronary artery bypass surgery (a technique which has not yet proved to be effective). The health professions must recognize these preventive techniques and be able to deliver them to the population in an effective manner.

Further, health administration can better recognize its responsibilities to and its influence on its own community's health. Thus, employment policies should consciously encourage health within the community. This may include active recruitment of staff from the neighborhood, on-the-job training, and other techniques that will use the tremendous power (financial, political, social, etc.) to improve the health of the community. The institution must also use its expertise and position to change other factors influencing health (accident prevention, alcoholism programs, support in housing, community organization, political action, and educational programs). This role also allows the health facility to become responsive to the needs of the community. The statesmen of health administration similarly may be helpful in altering national priorities.

Education in Health Administration

Another major concern in improving the health of Americans is the question of the distribution and education of health manpower. The maldistribution of quantity and quality of medical services in the urban ghettos and rural areas is well-known and needs no emphasis here.[34] The educational process for health administration should reflect the orientation toward health in the more positive sense as developed above.

First, we must reorder the priorities of medicine and the allied professions to recognize that health promotion and maintenance are at least as likely to produce health as are the disease oriented approaches so popular today. One must recognize that these preventive approaches include many unproven assumptions, but these are likely to be supported by the data as they accumulate. In the meantime, we must also recognize the infancy of health promotion in our medical culture without the glamour and excitement as depicted on television and without the more typical emotional, financial, and professional rewards of therapeutic medicine. These are apt to be less immediate than those of traditional curative health services, again for the many historical reasons.

To overcome this bias we suggest that the majority of the educational process must occur in new and different settings. Instead of the usual hospital environment, health administration students must be involved in community programs, particularly those involved with health maintenance. Because of the traditional lack of support in this area, financially, academically, politically and medically, it will require a commitment from student, teacher and consumer alike. The emphasis in these experiences will relate to health screening processes, health education, community participation, health maintenance and incidentally perhaps technology of the management of illness and disease.[35] It should be noted that the new educational setting alone will not necessarily accomplish a reorientation toward health issues. The sites selected for this field education must have established priorities for health promotion. Enhancement of this entire approach to education in health administration may be accomplished sooner and more practically by a requirement of meaningful participation in community health issues for accreditation.

Secondly, there should be direct involvement in health problems in the community, both for individuals and groups. An example of an individual problem may be that of a child with an abnormal blood lead level. The possible problems in this area of health promotion include the deprivation that preceded the pica, poor housing, increased lead in the air, poor access to medical care, social disorganization, poverty and certain later dysfunction, although there is no present illness. The educational process should allow learning regarding the complexities of dealing with the community agencies without the usual protection afforded by the hospital. For dealing with group issues, considerable understanding of biostatistics and epidemiology will be necessary, and these must continue to be part of the curriculum. However, the student must also become aware of and begin to deal with the very important confidentiality issues raised by the use of data banks both for the individual as well as for groups.

Third, the curriculum must include exposure to the new terminologies that will be developed relative to health. Since these are relatively unsophisticated at this point, the student of health administration should be involved in various approaches to health indices. In this regard there needs to be the continuing realization of the importance of living patterns on health. Certainly, it has been recognized for some time that cigarette smoking is related to dysfunctioning and death—coronary artery disease and lung cancer.[36] Other more subtle factors relating to health will become more apparent by identifying vulnerable individuals and groups. Belloc and Breslow have examined the relationship of various habits such as smoking, drinking, sleeping, exercising and eating. They have found that a clustering of "good" practices over a period of time is associated with longer life.[37] We must also be cognizant of the many changes in society and our environment that chronically or acutely affect the health of our citizens and include their impact in the health indices. For example, the technological advances of the last half century have contributed heavily to society's illnesses without apparent forethought: automobile use and air pollution, decrease in exercise and myocardial infarction, increased accidents, and now the energy crisis and cold; the stresses of today's pace and the problem of alcohol and drug abuse; the immorality of the war in Southeast Asia and increased teenage drop-outs and drug problems; the change in sex mores and present venereal disease epidemic; and on and on. These also must be entered into our equations of health and health promotion. Providers of health services must be constantly alert to the health implications of social and political change and anticipate them where possible.

In regard to such vulnerability, we will be challenged to develop the social, medical, economical and political forces to deal with the risk, once identified either in preventing dysfunction or at least in ameliorating it. One need only to recognize that we can identify now, even without newer sophisticated health terminology, that a baby born of a low socioeconomic mother is more apt to be of a lower birth weight, to have a higher mortality[38] and to suffer the unbearable consequences of not reaching his or her potential as a human being because of the effects of a relatively non-stimulating environment.[39] In addition, we must recognize the unusual demands that may make a person more vulnerable within his own familial or cultural environment. Thus, Green and Solnit have described the vulnerability of a child because of his family's responses to a critical illness.[40] Similarly, a culturally induced adaptive behavior may be maladaptive when put in the context of our larger society. In this regard we should recognize the positive features of various health practices within a culture (e.g., witch doctor) and incorporate these into our own.

Fourth, the education in the field must include better techniques to communicate with groups of people, to influence their behavior relative to health, that is health education. If not a role of the health administrator, at least he will have to have a firm understanding of this area in order to support it fully. We must be able to explain concerns about living patterns to people in a meaningful way. The most obvious first step is the strong health advocacy stance that we suggest is needed for health maintenance to move forward. This obviously means that all members of society must have free access to health maintenance (and hopefully to illness care as well). Furthermore, we suggest a strong effort to recruit students into the health administration field with a strong background in and motivation toward social change. This would include appropriate identification and support of disadvantaged students, thus creating a mixture of students of different backgrounds. The educational environment with this varied type of student would further improve the abilities for communication across cultures and hopefully stress the impact of life patterns on health and functioning. This suggests an educational focus beyond the teaching of methodological skills; it means a capacity to view programs in the light of their social significance and it means trying to teach students to anticipate the future and not to be tied to the past—no mean educational objective!

Fifth, the educational process must include involvement with long-range research problems of health. Since many of the social and environmental effects on health occur over prolonged periods of time, the health administrator of the future will need to understand the difficulties in the methodology and implementation of long-range research. Certainly, he will need to be concerned about effectiveness and efficacy in the broad sense developed by Cochrane.[41] Also, he will need to keep the goals of society and those of medical technology clearly separate. For example, even though medical technology has created the capability of treating quite well the congenital anomaly, meningomyelocele, Lorber at least has raised the very important issue of the quality of life that has been saved as well as the cost of that effort on the family and society.[42] Hopefully, the outcome measures of many of the long-range projects will include the more global approach to health and the role that various paraprofessionals may reasonably play in improving health and deciding the health goals.

Sixth, management and planning principles must be included in the curriculum. Many questions remain in regard to the issues of deployment of health professionals, the desirable size of health maintenance organizations, the relationship of health groups to public and private review organizations[43] and other problems related to bureaucracy. New methods of promoting health should be explored within the curriculum to deal with the changes created by the different population age and the different problems. For instance, the ability to alter behavior to suit society, as by psychosurgery and drugs, has raised significant questions regarding the goals of behavior modification.[44,45] What approaches should we take in this area? Also, the attempt to look at quality care under public or private auspices suggests to some creation of a mean level of care that will produce over-all mediocre health care.[46] Thus, the health administrator will need to assist in developing methods to deliver health care and to assess health and health care delivery.

Finally, and perhaps most important, the health administrator must learn those qualities that will allow him to orchestrate the groups necessary to promote health. For this, he will have to have a firm understanding of group dynamics involving consumers and providers as equals. This, with an appropriate use of and evaluation of financial approaches, will be necessary to develop health goals and also to implement programs. Thus, in humanizing people's health the choices may become ethical or societal and not as clearly clinical or scientific.[47] This does not belittle the importance of the professional consultant, be he economist, sociologist, physician, environmentalist, or other, but emphasizes the decision-making role of the consumer as well and recognizes the need for someone to fill the unique role of putting the puzzle together. There may be real confrontations between what is felt desirable for health and what the provider feels is quality care for illness. We must recognize the responsibility to keep our institutions open to new problems and new solutions, in this instance with health as our goal—the health of the individual and of society.

John Gardner has said "There are kinds of excellence—very important kinds—that are not necessarily associated with the capacity for self-renewal. A society that has reached the heights of excellence may already be caught up on the rigidities that will bring it down. An institution may hold itself to the highest standards and yet already be entombed in the complacency that will eventually spell its decline.

We are beginning to understand the processes of growth and decline in societies. We understand better than ever before how and why an aging society loses its adaptiveness and stifles creativity in its members. And we are begining to comprehend the conditions under which a society may renew itself. Renewal is not just innovation and change. It is also the process of bringing the results of change into line with our purposes."[48]

Notes

1. Michael L. Dolfman. "The Concept of Health: An Historic and Analytic Examination." *Journal of School Health,* October 1973. Vol. 43. pp. 491–497.
2. Howard Brody. "The Systems View of Man: Implication for Medicine, Science and Ethics." *Perspectives in Biology and Medicine,* Autumn 1973. Vol. 17. pp. 71–92.
3. Edward H. Kass. "Infectious Diseases and Social Change." *Journal of Infectious Diseases,* January 1971. Vol. 123. pp. 110–114.
4. William H. Stewart. "Health Assessment." Boisfeuillet Jones, ed. *The Health of Americans.* Englewood Cliffs, N.J.: Prentice Hall, 1970. p. 39.
5. Duncan W. Clark and Brian MacMahon. *Preventive Medicine.* Boston: Little, Brown & Co., 1967. p. 28.
6. Innes H. Pearce and Lucy H. Crocker. *The Peckham Experiment: A Study in the Living Structure of Society.* London: George Allen and Unwin, Ltd., 1943. p. 12.
7. G. Lamm. "Problems in the Definition of Ill Health." *International Journal of Epidemiology,* 1972. Vol. 1. pp. 356–359.
8. Constitution of the World Health Organization. *World Health Organization:* Basic Documents, 23 ed. Geneva: 1973. p. 1.
9. "Health Statistics Today and Tomorrow: The Report of the Committee to Evaluate the National Center for Health Statistics." *American Journal of Public Health,* October 1973. Vol. 63. p. 907.
10. Julius B. Richmond and Seymour L. Lustman. "Total Health—A Conceptual Visual Aid." *Journal of Medical Education,* May 1954. Vol. 29. pp. 23–30.
11. Innes H. Pearce and Lucy H. Crocker. p. 13.
12. Henry E. Sigerist. *The University at the Crossroads.* New York: Henry Schuman, 1946. p. 127.
13. S. Fanshel. "A Meaningful Measure of Health for Epidemiology." *International Journal of Epidemiology,* 1972. Vol. I .pp. 319–337.

14. Lester Breslow. "A Quantitative Approach to the World Health Organization Definition of Health: Physical, Mental and Social Well-being." *International Journal of Epidemiology,* 1972. Vol. I. pp. 347–355.
15. R. N. Rosser and V. C. Watts. "The Measurement of Hospital Output." *International Journal of Epidemiology,* 1972. Vol. I. pp. 361–368.
16. A. W. Grogona and D. J. Woodgate. "Index for Measuring Health." *Lancet,* November 6, 1972. Vol. 1. pp. 1024–1026.
17. S. B. Goldsmith. "The Status of Health Status Indicators." *Health Services Reports,* 1972. Vol. 87. p. 212.
18. S. Fanshel and J. W. Bush. "A Health Status Index and Its Application to Health-services Outcomes." *Operations Research,* 1970. Vol. 18. p. 1021.
19. F. I. Mahoney and D. W. Barthel. "Functional Evaluation: The Barthel Index." *Maryland Medical Journal,* 1965. Vol. 14. p. 61.
20. S. Fanshel. op. cit. p. 324.
21. A. L. Cochrane. "The History of the Measurement of Ill Health." *International Journal of Epidemiology,* 1972. Vol. I. 89–92.
22. Richmond and Lustman. Op. cit.
23. Fanshel. op. cit.
24. Breslow. op. cit.
25. "Health Statistics Today and Tomorrow: The Report of the Committee to Evaluate the National Center for Health Statistics." *American Journal of Public Health,* October 1973. Vol. 63. p. 891.
26. A. L. Cochrane. *Effectiveness and Efficiency: Random Reflections on Health Services.* Abington, Berkshires: Burgess & Son, Ltd., 1972.
27. H. G. Mather, et al. "Acute Myocardial Infarction: Home and Hospital Treatment." *British Medical Journal,* 1971. Vol. 3. p. 334.
28. Stephen A. Falk and Nancy F. Woods. "Hospital Noise-Levels and Potential Health Hazards." *New England Journal of Medicine,* 1973. Vol. 289. pp. 774–781.
29. Marshall H. Klaus and John H. Kennell. "Mothers Separated from Their Newborn Infants." *Pediatric Clinics of North American,* 1970. Vol. 17. pp. 1015–1037.
30. Antony Shaw. "Dilemmas of 'Informed Consent' in Children." *New England Journal of Medicine,* 1973. Vol. 289. pp. 885–890.
31. Raymond S. Duff and A. G. M. Campbell. "Moral and Ethical Dilemmas in Special Care Nursery." *New England Journal of Medicine,* 1973. Vol. 289. pp. 890–894.
32. Franz J. Ingelfinger. "Bedside Ethics for the Hopeless Case." *New England Journal of Medicine,* 1973. Vol. 289. pp. 914–915.
33. Norman W. Aznick, Steven M. Shannell and John J. Witle. "Benefits Due to Immunization Against Measles." *Public Health Reports, 1969.* Vol. 84. pp. 673–680.
34. John C. Norman, ed. *Medicine in the Ghetto.* New York: Appleton-Century, Crofts, 1969. pp. 1–10.
35. Kerr L. White, Jane H. Murnaghan and Clifton R. Gans. "Technology and Health Care." *New England Journal of Medicine,* 1972. Vol. 287. pp. 1223–1227.

36. E. C. Hammond. "Life Expectancy of American Men in Relation to Their Smoking Habits." *Journal of the National Cancer Institute,* 1969. Vol. 43. pp. 951–962.
37. N. Belloc and L. Breslow. "Relationship of Physical Health Status and Health Practices." *Preventive Medicine,* 1972. Vol. I. pp. 409–421.
38. Helen C. Chase, ed. "A Study of Risks, Medical Care, and Infant Mortality. *American Journal of Public Health.* (supplement), 1973.
39. Julius B. Richmond. "Disadvantaged Children: What Have They Compelled Us to Learn." *Yale Journal of Biology and Medicine,* 1970. Vol. 43. pp. 127–144.
40. M. Green and A. J. Solnit. "Reactions to the Threatened Loss of a Child: A Vulnerable Child Syndrome." *Pediatrics,* 1964. Vol. 34. p. 58.
41. Cochrane. op. cit.
42. J. Lorber. "Early Results of Selective Treatment of Spina Bifida Cystica." *British Medical Journal,* October 27, 1973. Vol. 4. p. 201.
43. Claude E. Welch. "Professional Standards Review Organization-Problems and Prospects." *New England Journal of Medicine,* 1973. Vol. 289. pp. 291–295.
44. Anne B. Somers. "PSRO: Friend or Foe." *New England Journal of Medicine,* 1973. Vol. 289. pp. 321–322.
45. Lawrence C. Kolb. "Psychosurgery-Justifiable" *New England Journal of Medicine,* 1973. Vol. 289. pp. 1141–1142.
46. William H. Sweet. "Treatment of Medically Intractable Mental Disease by Limited Frontal Leukotomy – Justifiable?" *New England Journal of Medicine,* 1973. Vol. 289. pp. 1117–1125.
47. Brody. op. cit. p. 85.
48. John Gardner. *Self-renewal: The Individual and the Innovative Society.* New York: Harper & Row, 1964.

Generic Versus Specialist Aspects of Health Administration*

The Commission's charge to the author was "to develop a new approach to education for health administration, that addresses the issues associated with the generic versus specialist aspects of health administration." The charge further specified that the educational model to be presented "push feasibility." At the outset, it should be noted that since 1970 the author has been engaged in the development of such a model at the University of Washington in Seattle. Much of what follows is based on the conceptualization and initiation of the Washington program.

Health Administration as a Specialty

Following the lead of Austin, this paper is concerned with the educational preparation of organizational executives who aspire to serve as directors of the variety of institutions and agencies concerned with planning for or delivery of health services.[1] As such, education for health administration is concerned with preparation for a tremendous diversity of potential assignments ranging from the management of very large and complex delivery organizations, offering one of the most challenging and difficult management assignments in our society, to quite small agencies with narrowly defined and limited objectives.

The practice of health administration may be viewed as having unique characteristics attributable to the highly individualized nature of the services provided, the dominance of the medical profession, coupled with the wide range of professionals of lower status, and the pluralistic nature of the health services industry.[2] The unique features of the practice of health administration have long been recognized and form the basis of specialized approaches to education. There has

* by William C. Richardson.

been some confusion, however, with respect to whether health administration is a specialty of the health professions or a specialty of administration.

Traditionally, a primary characteristic of the health professional has been a concern for welfare of the client, typically on a one-to-one basis, while the concern of management has been for the welfare of organizations and, particularly in public administration, the welfare of communities or groups of constituents. In this context, health administration is clearly a specialty of administration and its underlying disciplines and methods. Health administration seeks to apply these to a particularly complex service industry. Because of the pervasive and central role of administration in the health services establishment, however, it is useful up to a point to think of health administration as a specialty within the health care system. For example, this approach lends emphasis to the fact that health administrators represent but one component of the manpower complex required to deliver health services. Thus, it may be useful to talk about the health administrator as a health care specialist in order to emphasize his integral role in the system and the importance of health care as a component of his professional education. But fundamentally, the success of the health administrator in achieving beneficial results for his major constituencies will depend on his expertise with respect to administrative imaginativeness, ingenuity, and stature.

This is not to say that there is no place for health professionals in health administration. Having the professional knowledge of a physician or nurse in addition to management training or experience can be a very effective combination providing that the socialization process leading to primary emphasis on one-to-one relationships does not dominate. The identification with administration should be one's primary endeavor, with the health profession identification being secondary. The distinction can best be summarized by thinking of the differences between a physician who knows something about administration versus an administrator who is also a physician.

Turning to the question of the generic content of health administration: practice is based on an understanding of social organization and human behavior, economic relationships, and political processes, coupled with a working knowledge of specific methodology such as planning, budgeting, accounting, and quantitative methods. These categories of knowledge are presented in the broadest possible terms at the University of Washington, because the particular approach to or weighting of content areas under the broad headings depends to a considerable degree on the probable nature of the agency or institution in which the health administrator will be found. For example, the administrator of a general hospital can probably function more effectively with a thorough understanding of organization theory, particularly human behavior within organizations. On the other hand, the director of a relatively small community health agency is more likely to benefit from an understanding of other aspects of social organization, particularly human ecology and community organization.

Beyond the areas of knowledge that are fundamental to administration generally, there is an increasing body of knowledge peculiar to the health field which should be familiar to all health administrators. Included would be a working knowledge of various types of health programs, agencies, and institutions; an understanding of methods of organization, financing, and control of personal and community health services; and the contributions of the basic disciplines of social organization, economics, and political processes that deal directly with the health field.

While there are certainly generic aspects of health administration, there is also a strong tendency for health administrators to specialize with respect to the type of agency or institution which they manage, and for there to be little lateral career mobility. The latter is attributable to at least three factors. First, the individual must invest a considerable part of his career in learning the intricacies of a particular type of health institution or agency. In some cases this may include prior specialty training in one of the health professions as in the case of mental hospitals. Having developed a special body of knowledge from experience, there is a tendency to remain specialized. Second, formal education for health administration in different settings has itself been quite compartmentalized. It is not unusual to find several programs at a single university training individuals to become health administrators. Third, and perhaps as a result of the first two, there is considerable evidence of professional jealousy, suspicion, and, in some cases, inherent conflict between types of agencies and institutions. As will be noted below, this fragmentation may be less evident in the future.

The specialized knowledge that leads to identification with a particular type of institution or agency may be divided into three categories: knowledge or skills associated with the internal management of complex organizations; specialized analytic methods; and factors directly associated with the service being rendered.

Considering the first category, an obvious distinction is made in the requirements for the management of organizations differing in size and complexity. As these factors increase, personnel, service planning, and quality control became increasingly systematized and their coordination more formalized. Health administrators vary as a function of at least education and experience with respect to their ability to manage the more complex internal systems.

The second area of specialized knowledge, analytic methods, unlike the first, is not necessarily related to size or complexity of the organization, but rather may result from its mission. In the case of organizations whose function is the delivery of personal health services, only larger organizations can support, in the cost effectiveness sense, sophisticated analytic techniques such as operations analysis. However, formal analysis may represent an important service of smaller community health agencies. For example, in public health agencies, facility with the concepts and techniques of demography and epidemiology is essential to the health administrator. Similarly, the administrator of a medical care foundation must be adept at employing systematized exception reporting built on the notion of stochastic processes, an approach which offers the opportunity to identify the more serious problems, while avoiding the costs of fruitless data dredging.

Lastly, health administrators in different types of organizations or agencies develop special knowledge about the nature of the services rendered. This knowledge may include characteristics and needs of particular classes of patients (e.g., nursing homes); typical fiscal or organizational arrangements (e.g., health departments); applicable medical technologies (e.g., hospitals); or particular legal mandates or restrictions (e.g., mental health facilities). Consider, for example, the differences in required specialized knowledge between the administrator of an acute hospital and a nursing home administrator responsible for a facility of equal bed size. Even in a relatively small hospital, there is a wide range of technologically complex services, with the associated mixture of professional personnel and financial intricacies. The psychological and social well-being of the patient, while of some importance, is not the primary concern. The patients are not exposed to the hospital setting long enough for it to be a problem.

The same cannot be said for the nursing home, where the psychological and social health of the patients may be as important as their physical well-being. Further, the administrator's role in the nursing home, as in the mental hospital, seems to require a much more sophisticated understanding of the patients' illnesses and of factors influencing these illnesses than is the case for the administrator of an acute hospital.

In part this is true because the long-term care administrator can have a direct and important impact on the physical and social environment in which the patient lives over a prolonged period. In addition, however, the administrator rather than a group of attending physicians often has responsibility for establishing the expectations with respect to the range and quality of professional and other services to be made available.

To summarize, the author views health administration as a specialty of administration in the sense that practice represents primarily the application of the social and management sciences to a particularly complex service industry. The complexity of the health services establishment, as well as its size, justify relatively extensive formal preparation for the specialty and also have lead to marked subspecialization.

Struggling with Pluralism

Current developments in health services in the United States represent an effort to cope better with a number of underlying and quite persistent problems. Two of these problem areas seem particularly pertinent in terms of future requirements for health administration. First, medicine's growing complexity and the resultant specialization of services have had a profound influence on both the types of services that are most readily available and the degree of coherence among them. Specifically, it has become increasingly difficult for patients to find a suitable source of care when their problems are of a complex, ill-defined or not obviously serious nature. With specialization has come an increasing problem of coordination and continuity from the patient's perspective. If the patient has developed a relationship with a physician who provides primary care, specialist or not, there generally exists a little recognized but well developed referral network. This network is often patterned by hospital medical staff affiliations. Without an appropriate point of entry into this system, the patient must take his chances on correctly matching physician to complaint. But even for patients who have a point of entry, a retrospective examination of the overall care rendered patients for even moderately complex conditions often reveals considerable illogic in terms of medical management, unrelieved patient anxiety and unnecessary expense to both the patient and financing agencies.

The structuring and consequences of existing incentives within the health field in the United States represent the second problem area increasingly mentioned in the public debate over the organization of health services. This problem is one that transcends most others and whose resolution will have important implications. It is important to note that most of the services rendered by physicians, hospitals, and other providers are a result of patterns of illness and professionally agreed upon methods of diagnosis or treatment. It is only within this framework that financial and other incentives can modify the behavior of both provider and consumer.

If we think of the patient as seeking the effective diagnosis and management of a complaint rather than seeking a particular service such as an operation or an X-ray, then we see that the physician has a wide range of potential approaches to managing the complaint. In particular, given the appropriate set of resources and organizational framework, he may be able to handle the condition in equally satisfactory ways but with substantial variation in cost. In the traditional system, there is considerable incentive for a physician faced with a choice to hospitalize the patient. By doing so, he assures himself that the patient will receive continuous attention, have readily available a variety of ancillary services, and further, the patient will feel that he is receiving the best care. Under different systems, however, the same complaint might be handled by greater dependence on out-of-hospital services at less cost, with the savings accruing to both providers and consumers. Similarly, in the management of a long-term illness, there is little incentive for the physician to keep the patient "well" and out of the hospital under the current arrangement.

Turning to hospitals and their incentives, a most critical factor for a hospital is attracting competent physicians who will subsequently admit patients. There are a number of factors which make a particular hospital more or less attractive to a physician, but one is the availability of a wide range of services in his area of interest. Competition among hospitals in general and for medical staff members in particular has been one of the most costly competitions in the health field in the United States.

As a consequence of several problem areas, but particularly the two mentioned above, we have observed the emergence of three factors which have major implications for health administration. The first is the trend towards new organizational forms for the delivery of health services. The second factor is a market increase in the emphasis being placed on public accountability with respect to almost all facets of health services. The third factor is related to the first two, and indeed may be a consequence of them; namely, the conscious development of both governmental and voluntary entities charged with strategic as opposed to operational decision making responsibility which are quite distinct from delivery organizations.

Considering first new organizational forms for the delivery of health services, the federal government is pursuing a policy, including the encouragement of health maintenance organizations, which points toward substantially greater levels of organization and management in the health services establishment. Several proposals, including the health maintenance organization idea, imply a single source of responsibility for all of the patient's health needs. By incorporating an individual into a health delivery system, whether or not he is sick at the time, a defined point of access is provided with a formalized, contractual responsibility which has not, up to this time, existed for most of the population.

Apart from the health maintenance organization strategy, numerous efforts to reformulate the organization of health services have occurred over the past few years. For example, concern for access opportunities for the poor has resulted in the development of neighborhood health centers funded by government and free clinics staffed on a voluntary basis. Similarly, the demand on hospital emergency rooms and outpatient departments, which has increased dramatically over the past few years, has resulted in hospitals devoting more attention and resources to organized ambulatory care; competition among hospitals for high commitment on the part of medical staff members has led to the construction of adjacent medical practice buildings; concern for the adequacy of care rendered to rural populations has led to a variety of affiliation agreements between larger and smaller hospitals; and economic pressures have led to a wide range of shared services programs. The thrust of all of these organizational forms is towards integration either by formally relating ambulatory care and various types of institutional care, as in the case of health maintenance organizations; or by relating similar types of care as in the case of hospital affiliations. Both developments imply larger organizations with more comprehensive objectives, and, particularly in the case of the former, greater organizational demands being placed on the physician.

The second factor emerging from the problems listed earlier is that of increased public accountability. In addition to new delivery forms, we have witnessed in the United States a marked increase in the demand for systematic information concerning the operation of the system and for corrective mechanisms outside of these delivery organizations. With total expenditures for personal health services about $100 billion and with these expenditures concentrated to a considerable degree in the hands of government and large buyers of health insurance, increasingly the question is being raised as to whether or not the public is getting all that it should for the money spent. Representatives of the public in the form of elected officials, labor leaders, and others, are no longer willing to take appropriateness of utilization, quality of care, decisions on capital expenditures, and the desirability of certain methods of organization for granted. More and more providers are being required to justify their actions through formal analysis.

In the area of appropriateness of utilization, for example, we have moved very rapidly from a relatively innocuous federal requirement for hospital utilization review committees under the Medicare program to experimentation with concurrent utilization review systems designed to identify particular patients on a "real time" basis who may be using services inappropriately. In the area of medical care assessment, we have moved equally rapidly from a relatively limited focus or retrospective analysis of the appropriateness of surgical procedures and the completion of medical records to implementation, on a community-wide basis, of standards of care for a variety of diagnoses to be applied to ambulatory as well as inpatient care.

Beyond this, we have seen the recent development of numerous mechanisms, both voluntary and governmental, to bring the public into and/or to systematize decisions relating to costs, charges, and capital expenditures. Several states have established rate commissions and there is a strong trend towards requiring prior authorization by public authorities for construction of facilities and the addition of services.

Turning to the third factor, a desire to monitor new forms of delivery and the need for organizational settings within which mechanisms for public accountability may operate have led to the emergence of a greatly expanded segment of the health care field not directly concerned with either financing or delivery of services, but rather with their monitoring and coordination. Most conspicuous among these, although by no means the only entity, are health planning agencies. At the local level, the health planner is charged with the responsibility of balancing a multiplicity of often conflicting local interests in his attempt to identify societal and professional goals, of applying analytical capabilities to essentially technical questions ranging from ecological interrelationships to physician referral systems, of developing a plan or set of interrelated plans, and of serving as an effective change agent. In state government, the health planner in addition to working with local efforts, and reviewing and negotiating various intergovernmental arrangements, may also assume certain regulatory, resource allocation, and public policy functions within the broad area of health.

To summarize, the greatly increased complexity of the health services establishment, rapidly increasing costs, and public apprehension about the directions in which existing sets of arrangements and incentives are leading us have increased pressure for new forms of organization and additional public accountability. We are seeing the emergence of a new overlay of coordinative and monitoring activity whose management will require individuals with sound training as well as political adroitness.

Education for health administration to a greater degree than in the past must provide future administrators with an understanding of a wide variety of delivery organizations and agencies, and the way they function, in order to encourage awareness of the options for integration and coordination. Beyond this, health administrators must be prepared for much more intricate working relationships between the private and public sectors, as well as between what we have called the operational and strategic levels. Included would be expanded skills in "accounting" for and justifying current and proposed services. Finally, the political processes underlying the public policy framework within which health services are financed and delivered form an increasingly important area of study.

Developing an Educational Model

In light of the specialized nature of health administration and the developments in health services outlined above, several basic questions arise with respect to the design of formal educational opportunities for individuals who will occupy managerial roles in the system. To what degree should training for various managerial careers within health services be differentiated with respect to level of education and specialty content? To what degree should professional education occur in the academic setting as distinct from the work setting? Is there a preferred academic unit within which to locate management education for health services? And most importantly, what should be taught? The author's position with respect to these questions will be evident from the description of the educational model, but a preliminary summary may prove useful.[3]

With respect to the first question, the differentiation of levels and types of education, the goal should be to minimize fragmentation while still recognizing the real and well established difference in requirements for the practice of health administration discussed earlier. Given the generic aspects of health administration and the potential for future lateral career mobility, undergraduate and master's level education for health administration should differ more in intensity than in kind. Smaller and less complex practice settings, such as many nursing homes and ambulatory care clinics, do not demand the master graduate. Nevertheless, the same range of academic content, dealing with both administration and health services, is required. In contrast, master's level and doctoral level education in the health service field should differ in kind. The master's is the terminal degree for the professional practice of health administration. Doctoral level education is intended to serve quite different needs including basic disciplinary and applied research, as well as policy analysis in support of efforts to change the framework of constraints and incentives within which health services organizations and health professionals conduct their affairs.

Turning to the question of educational specialization by type of organization or agency (mission), the phenomenon of separate educational programs seems most undesirable. Apart from the fact that separate programs represent an excessively costly use of scarce faculty resources, separate programs do not represent an effective response to the trends discussed earlier. Within a hospital, a junior administrative person needs to be exposed, over time, to the operation of the many elements of the institution so that as his level of responsibility increases, he will have a firm understanding of the multiple implications of his decisions. When one moves beyond the single institution, however, the analogous need for experience with the various components of health services delivery is not so readily met. Part of the solution is to expose the individual as a student to substantial material covering the rationale and operation of all elements of the system. A program comprised of a mixture of faculty and students concentrating on different elements makes this possible.

The notion of a mixture of faculty who identify with various subspecialties of health administration is important. Types of organizations and agencies do have different goals, and the presence of sometimes conflicting advocacy by faculty is an important feature of the educational process.

Taking up the question of the degree to which preparation for a management career should take the form of formal course work, over the past several years health administration education has relied less on independent field training (such as the residency) and more on formal content. The reason is not that the field experience is deemed less valuable than it once was, but rather that there has been a rapid growth in the pertinent body of knowledge to be transmitted to students. Given a limited time period for formal education, this increased body of knowledge, the fruits of health services research, has been deemed relatively more valuable than supervised field experience and thus has displaced it to a considerable degree. Important efforts have been made to substitute field assignments that are concurrent with formal course work. Nevertheless, the student at graduation today is less well equipped for immediate administrative responsibility.

The phenomenon of increased formal content has also highlighted the fact that the curriculum need not directly reflect the knowledge and skills subsequently required for effective management practice. Some content can be learned more efficiently in a formal setting, while other aspects can only be learned on the job. For example, quantitative methods are expected to become increasingly useful to the manager, and should receive thorough treatment in the curriculum because of the difficulty of learning this material from experience. This is not to say, however, that understanding and making use of these technical skills will become the dominant ingredient of successful and effective management. Management will always be fundamentally a political process requiring a high level of interpersonal skills and adeptness at organizing and influencing groups with conflicting objectives.

The question of preferred academic location within a university for an educational program in health administration has been beaten around so much in educational circles over the past decades and its resolution is so dependent on specific university organization and resources that the author even hesitates to raise the issue. Nevertheless, if the objective is to minimize fragmentation in programs for health administration, while at the same time recognizing the legitimate need for some subspecialization as described earlier, provision must be made for a strong focus on the generic aspects of the specialty, health administration, while allowing diversity in the approach to the underlying disciplines and methods work.

At the University of Washington, this is accomplished by having a single university-wide degree program formally operated by a consortium of schools and departments through a faculty "group" whose chairman reports directly to the Dean of the Graduate School for purposes of the degree. At the same time, the Program's core faculty and the administrative location is in the Department of Health Services, School of Public Health and Community Medicine. This degree program (M.H.A.), including curricular, enrollment, and budgetary projections was considered as an independent entity for purposes of review and formal approval by the University's Board of Regents and the State's Council on Higher Education.

The key features of the University of Washington model reflect an approach to balancing the generic and specialist aspects of health administration. First, the Program is specifically designed to accommodate candidates whose career interests range across all types of organizations and agencies engaged in the delivery, coordinating, monitoring, or planning of health services. At the present time, for purposes of faculty advising, as well as funding, these interests have been grouped into three tracks: hospital administration; medical care administration; and health planning. In its developmental stage, the Program has concentrated on master's level education. Through collaborative arrangements with selected departments, doctoral students are soon to be enrolled, and serious consideration is being given to the development of an undergraduate track.

The curriculum for the master's level effort includes common distributional requirements for all students that incorporate the basic disciplines and the minimum of methods content that we feel underlie health administration practice in any setting. These may be classified as follows:

- Social and Organizational Theory.
- Intermediate Economic Theory, including applications to social policies and programs.
- Public Policy and the Political Process.
- A Tools or Methods requirement, incorporating quantitative methods, accounting or public budgeting, and planning methods.

Consistent with the tendency for students to have a more or less specialized career interest, the actual courses taken to satisfy these distributional requirements vary considerably. Students in the hospital administration track tend to satisfy most of their distributional requirements in the Graduate School of Business, closely following the first year of the MBA curriculum. Students in the medical care administration track take some course work in the business school, but are also inclined to take selected courses in the Department of Economics, the Graduate School of Public Affairs, and the Department of Urban Planning. Students in the third track take a heavier concentration of urban planning courses and take courses in areas such as statistics, social organization, and demography from arts and sciences departments.

It should be noted that close working relationships with the participating schools and departments must be maintained through the group mechanism in order to accomplish effective student counselling. Considerable effort goes into monitoring both the current content and apparent quality of a wide variety of courses. Detailed information is provided for faculty advisors during each quarter.

Beyond the distributional requirements, all students are required to satisfy a health services core which is provided for postdoctoral fellows, selected undergraduate medical students, a limited number of graduate students from elsewhere on campus, as well as the students enrolled in the health administration program. The core consists of one course each quarter for the six quarters that the student is on campus. The first year courses cover an introduction to health services, including the biological, behavioral, economic, and political processes underlying community and personal health services delivery as well as the specific financing, organization, and control of the wide range of planning and delivery activities in the field. The three courses offered during the second year of the program as part of the health services core are the applications of the basic disciplines to health services: medical sociology, medical economics, and the politics of health. By taking the health services core as a cohort, students have the opportunity over the two year period to interact with each other. In addition, there is substantial exposure to other health professionals, particularly physicians.

Finally, each track has associated with it specialized field experiences and concentration courses. For example, in the area of hospital administration students are placed in a supervised summer internship between the first and second year and complete an applied field analysis or research project keyed to a local institution during the second academic year. The concentration courses for hospital administration focus on elements of patient care, hospital law, medical staff organization, hospital finance, and applications of operations analysis. On the other hand, students in the medical care administration track, depending on specific interests, would be placed in a community health agency during the summer, undertake an applied research project, usually in an agency setting, and in their concentration courses would focus less on internal management of large delivery organizations, with more emphasis on community organizations, program planning and analysis, target population analyses, and prepayment financing.

To summarize, the educational model that has been developed at the University of Washington provides for all health administration education to be under a single program, and at any one level (i.e., baccalaureate or master's) to be under a single degree. The model recognizes that there is a set of disciplines and methods which underlie all health administration, but that the appropriate approach to teaching them varies as a function of the students' career direction. Medical care content and the application of the basic disciplines to health services is provided all students as a cohort, and with an opportunity to mix with students at various levels in the health professions. Specialty courses, student advising, field placement and supervision, and applied research advising is the responsibility of a core faculty who have academic interests directly related to the subspecialty or track within the program.

Faculty and Students

The faculty for the master's level group degree program are drawn from the School of Public Health and Community Medicine, the Graduate School of Business, the Graduate School of Public Affairs, the Department of Urban Planning in the College of Architecture and Urban Planning, the Departments of Economics, Sociology, and Geography in the College of Arts and Sciences, and the Health Sciences Schools of Medicine, Nursing, and Social Work. The group is comprised of 22 members, with the program director serving as chairman.

Members of the group have been selected on the basis of their interest in health services administration and planning, including contributions to health services research. The committee is envisioned as playing roles akin to that of directors, acting collectively on policy issues and serving individually as a link to their respective schools and departments. Since the beginning, student admissibility to the program has been subject to approval by not only the Department of Health Services, but also the other schools providing basic administration education.

The ongoing management of the program is in the hands of the core faculty. This group of four has its faculty appointments in the Department of Health Services, School of Public Health and Community Medicine. Each has interests and experience keyed to one of the tracks within the program. In addition to concentration courses, this faculty group offers about one-third of the health services core.

The remainder of the core, specifically the introduction to health services, medical sociology and the politics of health are offered by social science or community medicine faculty also appointed within the Department of Health Services but not directly affiliated with the Program in Health Services Administration and Planning.

Finally, some of the advantages of the model described above and some of the difficulties with it should be mentioned. Considering the advantages, this approach to health administration education provides the University an opportunity to be quite responsive to changes in demand for education to meet specific career interests within health administration more generally. Further, it is relatively easy to change the mix of specific courses used to satisfy distributional requirements as a function of career interests and changes in the quality of instruction within certain areas. Particularly in a time of scarce resources in higher education, the additional advantage of minimizing duplication of faculty offering work in the basic disciplines and methods areas is also an important consideration. Finally, the faculty most directly associated with the program are able to concentrate on the application of administration and planning to the health field in a setting in which specialty interests are well recognized, but isolation and fragmentation are discouraged.

Along with the advantages, the model of health administration education described has associated with it certain hazards. First, the approach is heavily dependent upon a mechanism for providing the core faculty current and accurate information with respect to course offerings in other academic units. Even with this information, the faculty member must devote considerable attention to individual student interests and goals, working to match these with the resources available. The model is designed for students who have fairly specific career objectives in mind. Nevertheless, there are students each year whose objectives change and for whom particularly careful counselling must be addressed. By the time, during the first year, that summer assignments are to be made the students must have established a fairly firm idea of the direction for the coming four quarters in order to get maximum benefit from the curriculum.

A second potential hazard is a weakening over time of the complex set of relationships that must exist at all levels of administration among the participating academic units. The venture depends on a University commitment and mechanism to channel the necessary resources into the participating units in rough proportion to the effort expended, as well as a strong identification by the units themselves with the health administration program. Careful management is obviously required.

Finally, consideration of the specialist versus generic aspects of health administration discussed earlier in the paper and the educational model proposed imply the desirability of educational programs for health administration being located on relatively large university campuses which include resources in at least the areas of health sciences, business administration, and public affairs, and preferably several additional resources. While there are many such settings within the United States, the climate for a university-wide collaborative effort as described has not developed in many of them. Where the potential exists, experience at the University of Washington would suggest that there are major advantages to the approach described and that the potential hazards can be avoided.

Notes

1. Charles J. Austin. "What is Health Administration?" Washington, D.C.: Commission on Education for Health Administration, October 1973.
2. Ibid. pp. 2–6.
3. The author considers the design and provision of continuing education opportunities of major importance. This subject, however, is left to another paper in the series.

The Future Health Administrator as Viewed by Others*

Current Attitudes Toward the Role of the Administrator

Very rarely have I read a plan for the future of our health care system that emphasizes or really talks about the health administrator or the need for one. I have not heard the administrator criticized for the ineffectiveness of the system—except, of course, by doctors. Is this proof of how insignificant he or she is thought to be? Listen to the Senator from Massachusetts, Edward Kennedy: "The system is riddled with waste and inefficiency, grossly uneven quality, highly inflated costs, and severe shortages of medical manpower."[1] Blue Cross Association President, Walter J. McNerney, alludes to the administrator in discussing Management by Objective, an approach widely used in business and industry: "Hospitals should take bolder leaps toward the concept. People are leaving the health field because they are bored administratively," he notes.[2] He views Management by Objective as an important managerial tool which might provide greater clarity about administrative functions and consequently greater commitment and involvement by administrative personnel.

Kerr L. White, professor of medical care and hospitals at John Hopkins University, in his provocative lead article in *Scientific American,* wrote: "What is clear is that containment of our overall health costs within tolerable limits will be difficult without expert management of those systems. At present our hospitals and health care institutions are largely run by amateurs with on-the-job training." He is referring to the fact that of 17,500 hospital administrators only one-third have had anything that could be regarded as formal training for "managing these complex organizations."[3]

* by Nathan J. Stark

These statements of two authorities reflect some of the problems and the promise of a new kind of involvement for health care administrators in emerging health care systems.

Anticipating the Arena for Administrators of the Future

It is essential that the Commission on Education for Health Administration, educators, and practitioners look ahead at least ten years or more to anticipate the kinds of systems, the nature of the environment, and the potential for a new and enlarged role for administrators that will be required in the health field. We can predict that the social and public services sector, of which health is a part, will be managed, financed, and delivered differently. We can probably anticipate other developments by 1980–1985 including the following:

1. There will be improved planning, coordination, and integration of social services generally, and we will have a better understanding of the relationship of housing, income, education, and employment to health status than we do today. These fields will be less isolated from one another, and we will have improved understanding of how to develop them in concert with one another.

2. There will be closer linkages, service relationships and communications systems among health care institutions than presently.

3. Principles of industrial management and organizational behavior will be better known in the health field and applied to ongoing systems.

4. Public representatives and consumer organizations will play a much larger role than presently in the design, control, and evaluation of health and other social services programs. Consumers will know more and be more demanding on their own behalf.

5. Rural health systems will be tied more closely to urban systems, with the latter serving as the major backup for the rural and smaller communities.

6. Emergency medical services will be available throughout most of the nation and will be provided with good backup support from large urban medical care centers.

7. Government will be a higher factor in financing, evaluating and establishing of service standards in the health field.

8. Physicians will function in larger group settings, and medical care foundations will continue to carry prestige.

9. Hospital and institutional trustees will be more heavily involved than ever in determining health policies, in determining the direction of the total institution, and in setting standards of care.

Impact on Administrators and Others

Without a doubt, the function of management will be more important than ever before. It will become—if it is not already—an essential commodity. Effective health administrators will be in short supply. Many of the current administrators will lack the experience, outlook, and training to qualify for the management tasks that lie ahead in the new health setting. Managers from other fields will enter the health arena and will partially fill the gap.

The role of management in the health field will be redefined, enlarged and strengthened, and restructuring of the management function will occur. Professional schools of health management will respond to changes and demands in society and a new kind of health administrator will emerge.

The Essential Need for the Management Function

Those of us who have been associated with management through the years are well aware of the central place and the essential need for managers in the operation of the major enterprises of our nation. This need for management stems from technological advances and scientific innovations, societal expectations, the immense size and degree of specialization in the labor force, and the mounting wealth and accumulation of resources in this country. Generally, management serves to translate or channel resources toward desirable goals and into deliverable consumer services and products. Management and managerial expertise become even more critical in a period of rapid change, such as the current energy crisis, an economic downturn, a sudden shift in social expectations, or the rapid buildup in health services.

Management serves an essential purpose in helping to interpret trends, translate needs and options to top level policy makers, design and establish systems, measure performance, and evaluate outcomes. It is to management that institutions (business and social service) look for help to formulate policy choice, to plan and carry out new programs, assist in establishing goals, and negotiating agreements and contracts, and even in suggesting worthy research projects and objectives.

Industrial Management as the Model

In business organizations we refer to the person or persons who bring people together for action and implementation as management. In non-profit organizations, such persons are generally called administration. Over the years each has created its separate art, technology, jargon, professional societies and professional schools. In some way or another—I leave this to others for historical verification—the term "management" projects an image of the more professional, successful, and adventurous activity. The term "administration" on the other hand, has become associated in health with inefficiency, waste and lack of responsiveness to its clients (the patients). We hear frequently today that since the non-profit institutions (and most of our health institutions come in this category) are under no obligation to show a profit, they are under no compulsion to keep a lid on costs. When one authoritative person refers to most hospital administrators as amateurs with on-the-job training, does this mean that administrators are different from the vast majority of business executives comprising our management group? It does not! Is there something unique, then, about an administrator in the health field compared to other management?

Health Service Administrators Compared to Business Managers

Cyril O. Shuler, writing for *Hospital Administration,* states that while many academicians hold tenaciously to the proposition that hospital administration is different from that of other management, the heads of health administration schools and and institutions are frequently stumped when asked what specifically is unusual about this field. Dr. Shuler points out, "In some health administration practices, there is little relation to accepted business and industrial practices. Others entwined in accepted rules of medical practice, can be viewed as illegal restraint, unfair competition, or discriminatory pricing practices in business or industry. A few of these factors ignore, or operate counter to accepted elementary economic principles." He points out some fifteen characteristics which are considered unique to health administration. These range from the patient, ". . . usually an involuntary user of the health institution," to the diversity of third-party payment rules, to the ease with which mistakes or poor decisions can be covered, to the more humanistic needs of rendering quality service, to how the patient pays for care and how he is charged for such care and then to the free market aspects of our society in which Dr. Shuler points out the health field is a monopoly. He also alludes to the dichotomy existing between boards of directors and the medical staff on the one hand and administration on the other. And finally there are the "moral and ethical issues of health service" that the administrator must face.[4]

Dr. Shuler does not assert the absence of these same factors elsewhere in our economy, but does state that the combination of similar factors is not found in administrative activities outside the health field. His thesis, therefore, is that the net effect of these factors creates a need for specialization in health skills and knowledge, not required in other vocations.

The characteristics which Dr. Shuler considered to be unique may be so in combination, but every business faces to some degree the same problems and obligations.

Perhaps, the lack of controls—public or governmental—over our health institutions has created a condition which puts the administrator under an unusual obligation for the protection of his patients' interests. In business, through consumer protection laws, there is not only the moral but legal obligation to look out for their customers' interests. The characteristics of health administration in most instances overlap with business—especially in the area of economics.

Peter F. Drucker asserts that the service institution is not very different from a business enterprise. "It faces similar challenges in seeking to make work productive. Nor does the service institution differ very much from business enterprise in respect to the manager's work and job, and in respect to organizational design and structure, or even in respect to the job and structure of top management."[5] Drucker goes on to point out that the service institution is different in respect to its purpose, values, objectives, and ultimate contributions to society.

Measuring Performance and Outcomes of Service Institutions

Stockholders and directors keep the pressure on management to show a profit, to grow and to get a greater share of the market. Business organizations effectively use the principles of management, control and evaluation. They use such disciplined tools as technology transfer, management by objectives, budgeting, long-range planning, profitability accounting, and incentive techniques. Generally, firms that use these programs are the more aggressive and successful ones.

By this measure we might think of the health institution as one of the less aggressive businesses. One writer, H. Igor Ansoff, in *Management In Transition* says of this non-profit less aggressive organization that it differs from the more aggressive profit-making firm in that the latter uses objectives as a management tool; whereas, the former uses "common process" (e.g., curing patients). Ansoff states further that "because non-profit organizations are process oriented, and because they lack quantitative measurements and techniques for evaluating outcomes, the performance discipline is usually lax and much less rigorous than in the busines firm."[6] Drucker confirms these findings and states that service institutions have failed to measure and evaluate performance and then act on the basis of the findings. Our health institutions have thus lagged behind the business firm in effectiveness and strength. Can our non-profit agency learn from our business firms? Some of the programs we might look to are management by objectives, incentives, vastly improved accounting to identify and quantify costs, management techniques to reduce overtime, improve working conditions, and make maximal use of industrial engineers, systems analysts, automatic machines and computers. All help to keep costs down. The administrator must be compelled to justify his existence and performance not only in the economic sense, but in terms of social profitability or fulfilled human needs.

Problems to Overcome in Assigning a New Role to the Health Administrator

There are several problems and limitations to be overcome before it will be possible to give substance to a new role for and definition of the function of a manager in the health fields.

Present Role a Highly Circumscribed One

The present health services administrator is seen as an individual with a limited scope of responsibility, usually restricted to technical and more routine tasks within an institution or an agency. He lacks an entrepreneurial image altogether. In some critical aspects of ongoing institutional life he is excluded or instructed to refrain from any direct interference or involvement. The historical pattern has been that the administrator in health affairs has developed as a caretaker.

In my experience with the boards of three hospitals, trustees' perceptions of the role of the hospital administrator ranged between housekeeper and office boy, unless he happened to have an M.D. after his name. Then he was generally thought to be misusing his talent on administrative work.[7]

Try to persuade almost any group of medical men that they should not be running our hospitals. Two doctors, one from the far west, the other from the eastern seaboard responding independently to the question of doctors' attitudes toward hospital administrators said, quite emphatically, "We have no use for them!" Now, part of this (I hope a good part) was tongue in cheek. But the response did represent what I have found among many M.D.'s, an antagonism for the guy in charge—particularly one whose knowledge of professional medical procedure may not be so great as their own.

A doctor who has the ear of a trustee can frustrate an administrator from carrying out effectively the very policy that the board of trustees has established. Respect, as pointed out earlier, of the board of trustees is not always present.

In my estimation any top administrator should be accorded the same treatment as for-profit corporations give their chief executives. The top administrator needs the security of having a voice in the policy councils in order to enunciate and carry out that policy. Using a corporate form of organization is more generally understood by businesmen and others on the boards of trustees and enhances the image of the administrator who is then recognized as the chief executive.

How the Management Role is Determined

Who defines and determines the function of management in the health sectors? Who legitimizes the role of the manager? How are the status relationships maintained, controlled, and enforced? Who determines "turf boundaries?" What is the process by which one professional participant in the health institution is able to control another?

There is a great deal of literature in the behavioral sciences which sketches out the dynamics of relationships of the key players and participants in the health game. The findings are well-known to all of us here. There are many persons, forces, and factors that determine the role and the function of the health administrator including physicians, trustees, other medical care professionals, scientific and professional societies, professional schools, public relations and news media, and society itself—and also his own self image. It is fair to say many managers are fulfilling the role expectations others have for them as caretakers and record keepers.

Conditions of change and pressures for solutions may accelerate the process of enlarging and strengthening the manager's involvement and range of responsibilities in the health field; perhaps, some of these expectations are changing. Trustees and physicians (two dominant forces in the local community) will be under increasing pressure to answer to community civic leaders and political figures, consumer organizations and professional groups (nurses, hospital accountants, et al.) regarding the nature, acceptability and inadequacies of existing health systems. The principal participants will see management in a new light and as a responsible and useful mode in helping resolve major difficulties and preventing breakdowns in the health care delivery system field.

Small Size of Most Health Institutions

Most health institutions and organizations in the typical community are quite small. It is unusual for a health administrator to supervise more than several hundred employees. In Kansas City, for example, the local head of TWA or Bell Telephone will be responsible for over six thousand employees. The largest hospital in Kansas City will not employ two thousand persons. The health field is characterized by a myriad of small, semi-autonomous entities and service units. The manager in such an environment tends to take a back seat compared to other managers in industrial and governmental enterprises.

However, all of this is changing because the many health organizations and service units are increasingly becoming interrelated and involved in a larger community process. I doubt that there is any way that this trend can or will be slowed down. Trustees of the larger institutions are working more closely together in sharing their services, planning of medical centers, eliminating duplicate facilities, and becoming more sensitive to the health consumer. Institutions are not losing their right of self-determination, but they are devoting much more energy to joint programming which will better serve the overall needs and interest of the community.

As new and larger social service systems and networks come into being, the various professionals find that they are able to institute cooperative systems for the creative involvement of all parties concerned. Moreover, as electronic systems are applied to the measurement and evaluation of outcomes, there will be a greater need than ever for cooperation among all of the diverse professional members functioning throughout the health sector.

One author in the management field has summarized this point well: "To serve greatly increased demands, to provide continuity of services over longer spans of time, to permit coordination of workers, to allow work on projects of larger size, to make possible greater use of expensive equipment, to centralize and perhaps automate administration of clerical work, to correlate professional work with other kinds of service—for all of these purposes it has become more feasible to administer prepayment for services on a large scale through a third party, to bring larger numbers of professional workers into a going organization as salaried adjuncts."[8]

The organization and work setting in health are increasingly complex and interrelated with other social service settings. There are few isolated work units and few autonomous workers; all touch and come in contact with larger organizational systems.

Rural Communities

Health service administrators in smaller communities and rural areas face problems of a different nature from their counterparts in the large metropolitan cities. The administrator in the small community is "isolated" in many ways. He lacks the financial and material resources that are taken for granted in larger health institutions. He views the metropolitan health administrators as closely linked with one another in a communications and technical support network that excludes the "outstate" and rural communities. He frequently works with board of trustees members and local leaders who have little real understanding of the changing character of the health system in America.

New Concept of What the Professions Can Be

A new image and role for the health manager can be facilitated by developing and promoting a concept of what the profession can be and what part the managers might play in the health field. This should be a joint responsibility and objective of professional associations and professional schools in the health field. There is no reason that the focus on functions, expectations, and performance of health managers cannot be sharpened and improved.

The Committee for Economic Development in its recent position statement on health has said, "The key to the success of the health system is its management. There has been little application to the field of health care of such managerial and administrative techniques, which are commonplace in business and industry."[9] Herman Somers has pointed out in a recent address, "The trend we have discussed—systemization, institutionalization, standards and control—among other developments, have placed a new premium on effective management, an ingredient which too long was conspicuously lacking in the health field."[10]

An Expanded Role and Function for the Health Administrator

As suggested in previous sections, we are entering a period when the health manager will have a whole new set of demands and expectations placed upon him. These forces will require an expanded role and function for the administrator. The outcome will be a restructuring and strengthening of the function of management in the health field. The increase in responsibilities for managers in health fields will be reinforced by philosophical positions taken by professional associations and as a result of new programs for professional education of health administrators.

BROAD AREAS OF PROFESSIONAL COMPETENCE

How might we describe the areas of competence of the new health manager? In broadest terms we can visualize his role and involvement as follows:

1. He must have an acute sense of what institutional life is like within his agency and how to deal with it effectively. The knowledge which he gathers regarding the institution becomes professionalized and operational through him. That is, he knows or learns the norms, expectations, performance levels, attitudes, plans and conflicts within the institution. He filters this data base through his professional expertise to the achievement of the larger goals of the institutions as well as to the objectives of key participants within and without the agency. He is an involved, listening, responding individual. He possesses some of the skills of the applied behavioral scientist which he is able to apply to group process, an aspect of institutional life which he regards as a critical element in performance.

2. He is an effective negotiator, listening post, diagnostician and counselor in relationships involving outside health provider institutions and agencies. He is a major source of information to his trustees

and policy makers in assessing the direction and requirements for change in institutional relationships.

3. The health manager is skilled in the use of task groups as they may be used both inside and outside his institution. He has the ability to create, utilize, guide and work with such groups. Normally, these will be temporary task or project teams. They will be comprised of multi-professional individuals, working under the guidance of a project manager. These groups will be a major source of information to him about the life within the institution, its direction and potential. Such groups will be instrumental in helping him find his way around the institution and the community.

4. He will be highly knowledgeable in the use of performance measurement techniques and electronic data systems. He will make use of the results and information derived from these systems to modify the design and structure of the institution.

5. The manager is experienced in dealing with government agencies and interpreting to them the priority needs of the community and of his own institution.

This idealized model of the new manager is alien to the notion of the administrator as an autonomous expert or resident consultant. I am positing an activist individual who is concerned with pulling together and integrating a knowledge base for the purpose of making it operational and useful in the ongoing life of the institution.

Evaluation of Institutional Purpose and Performance

Peter Drucker states that health service institutions must impose upon themselves the discipline of continually scrutinizing their purpose and performance. Clearly, the health manager will need to be adept and skilled in implementing a process for the continuing evaluation of the institution. Drucker indicates that the questions and areas of concern should focus upon the following.[11]

- The institution needs to answer the question, "What is our business and what should it be?"
- Clear objectives and goals should stem from the institution's definition of its primary mission.
- Priorities of concentration and need should determine the targets of the institution.
- The institution and the manager need to define measurements of performance.

- The institution needs to use these measurements to feed back on its efforts.
- There is need for an organized audit of objectives and results to hereby eliminate unsatisfactory activities and conditions.

He places the greatest emphasis upon the final point which relates to the quantitative measurement of results in determining whether the results justify a continuation or alteration of given activity.

Acceptance by Others of the New Role of the Manager

What view will others take of the new role and function projected for the health manager? Will the physicians, trustees, medical care professionals, consumer groups, civic and political leaders accept the manager's increasing involvement in the activities sketched out above?

It is possible that conditions will be such that there will be no choice except to support the deeper involvement of the manager. Unless other professional participants can invent better mechanisms for planning, policy development, resource allocations, budgeting, control, measurement and evaluation, then it will be necessary to rely upon the skilled, professional manager and his staff. There is nothing to prevent the various professional and technical staff members in the organization from participating in the various management and allocation systems.

There is no reason that they should be excluded from top level decision making responsibilities. Increasingly, professional and technical staff members throughout the institution will insist upon being cut in on the "action." But this, again, will add another task to the job of the manager—that is the task of designing, negotiating, and guiding the decision making process and structure within the institution.

Increased Responsibility for Management of Resources

As part of his enlarged responsibilities, the health administrator will have a great deal to say about the control and disposition of major resources of the institution. Among those resources will be:

- Budgets and budget allocations
- Distribution and use of most medical care and allied health manpower within the institution

- Contracts and contract negotiations with medical groups, medical care foundations, employee associations and unions

In looking after the institution's resources, the manager necessarily will be intimately involved with trustees, community policy makers, government agency heads, key medical care and professional persons and many others in positions to affect the decision making process. The manager's resources, then, will include not only men, money, and material but will embrace other less tangible considerations. His access to policy councils, his responsibility for negotiating major contracts, his intimate knowledge of life within the institution (including patients), his close contact with administrators and decision makers in other health institutions, his skill in the use of small task groups, his almost daily review of hard data relating to the performance of his institution and outside agencies, his interest and instinct to translate and use his knowledge within an operational context, reach consensus and make decisions—all of these must be counted as important resources of both a personal and professional character. Certainly they are the kinds of resources that are essential to healthy and continued life of a health institution.

CODES OF CONDUCT AND VALUE SYSTEMS

The evolution of the health administrator will find him increasingly confronted with conflicting demands and competing choices. His professional society and the professional schools in particular can and should provide him with some of the essential moral and philosophical underpinning in his personal makeup. There will be occasions when he will have to decide in effect who he really works for and on behalf of whose interest he is engaged: trustees, consumers, physicians, the overall community, unions—or even his ego needs. It will not be unusual for him to experience some confusion and self conflict. However, codes of professional conduct, value systems within society, and individual preferences will govern his choices ultimately in these instances.

USE OF APPLIED BEHAVIORAL SCIENCE

The behavioral scientist has frequently found the professional manager his most sympathetic partner. Few persons know better at firsthand the agonies, frustrations and joys of cooperative and organizational endeavor than managers. Few persons in society have a more genuine concern for diagnosing, easing and resolving human difficulties in organizational life than the behavioral scientist. His desire to help provide a foundation for a more creative and satisfying work environment does indeed parallel the objective of the manager.

Behavioral science will provide us with important tools in dealing with complex human service networks. The professional manager will welcome these tools and, in fact, will recognize that he cannot survive without them.

He will not be a mere technician or simply a skilled operator capable of implementing policies over which he has no control. He will indeed participate actively in the analysis and development of the policy itself, whether he works for HEW or OMB, state government, county and regional organizations, private industry, or a major health care institution. He will have a major concern for valued questions and frequently will ask both privately and publicly, "What is the best interest of the community?" He is concerned about technical considerations, "Is it feasible to carry out the policy or proposal?" He recognizes that he functions within an environment where personal, institutional and community needs and objectives are intertwined and related. It is little wonder that the health manager will find his job so fascinating and challenging.

Realistic Expectations of Professional Education to Develop Leaders

There are practical limits to what can be expected of professional schools in the preparation of young persons for careers in health management and in renewing and upgrading the levels of competence of present practitioners. By focusing for a moment on the nebulous nature of managerial leadership, we can perhaps sense boundaries between school and work place.

When considering leadership in institutional settings, I tend to think of organized cooperation. My concept of management leadership does not involve a traditional top down organization chart but rather an inverted chart where the leader serves those he leads. Cooperation, then, is the key word to successful leadership. Likewise, I do not subscribe to the tenet of so-called scientific management of a few years ago, that professionalism of administration is a repeatable technique. On the contrary, variety of experience plays a far greater role in leadership development. Merely being efficient through scientific management has had a built-in mechanism getting us to the wrong place in a big hurry. Look, for example, at the gruelling experience of war, pollution, energy crises, etc.

One who has never managed on his own will have a difficult if not impossible time learning how to do so in a classroom. That is why I earlier alluded to on-the-job training. Formal training in a classroom is a small part of the administrator's education. Most of it will of necesity take place on the job. Doctors from the beginning of their profession have as a part of their profession been teachers. Every executive should also be a teacher. A good part of his time must be spent in teaching as well as sharing with his colleagues his perception of the process in which they are working together. Here, then, we come back to what I consider the most vital part of leadership: cooperation. This is a teaching and learning process, getting others to understand what others are doing and why. This would not only help the young aspiring administrator but also would be effective in breaking down the barriers created by doctors and other health professionals to the administrator trying to accomplish his job.

The plain fact is that administrators are being developed right now without the benefit of formal development programs, and some administrators are being developed despite those programs.

I don't subscribe to "vestibule" training for managers. The artificial environment does not substitute for the real development that takes place on the firing line. How, for example, can you teach one to have the courage to take risks or to know whether it is wise to take such risks and then to have the willingness to accept responsibility? How do you teach the administrator when to face the fact that he must remain flexible in the face of this courage and sometimes modify or retreat from a decision without feeling he has lost face? It can only come about under real conditions, tested under fire. The more difficult situations the administrator faces, the more confidence he will gain—and confidence makes for more effective decision makers.

All of this does not preclude the need for knowing all there is to know about computer applications, finance, accounting principles, and so forth. These I classify as technology. Knowing the basics of one's field is absolutely essential. These are the tools of administration but they are not the end product of managing. Formal education and a liberal arts program certainly are valuable, but they only create a shortcut for some individuals through the management development process. Formal schooling is not a substitute for doing.

Now we are into the vicious circle syndrome. If on-the-job training is so important to administrative development, those at higher levels in the institution or agency must be strong and confident administrators. In addition they must not only have a desire to teach but the capability as well. As with any good teacher they must take time to work with students, point out and accept errors, and give guidance on future performance.

We have spoken about an organizational structure which is horizontal, rather than vertical where it would appear no one is in charge and everybody is partly in charge. Now, we talk about a concerned public who wants to belong to this organization to observe what is happening and to blow the whistle when they do not like what is going on. The administrator is going to be hard pressed to find ways of mobilizing the public outrage. There are many ways of doing this. One obvious but by no means easy way is to broaden community participation.

Citizens no longer have much hesitation in organizing to bargain collectively about the location of a health agency or hospital. Some have even gone so far as to take over a hospital in order to satisfy demands. There is a new pattern of leadership emerging in many communities which is breaking up leadership monopolies traditionally held by business men, lawyers and the early settlers. Any top executive whether he holds power within his organization or not must be impressed with the difficulty of getting anything done without involving the community. Internal power is a facade. As patients and would-be patients, the consumers will increasingly want to help make the key decisions that affect them. After all, they are the people affected and wonder why they should not, therefore, participate with the organization's managers in making those decisions.

A Proposed Educational Approach for Developing Health Administrators

Through the years, professional schools have been instrumental in training and channeling some very capable administrators in high-level positions.

It is worth noting that schools of business management and public administration are no longer dominated by a single academic discipline. Business schools have long since freed themselves from the domination of the economist, and public administration no longer takes its directions from political science. Instead, these two professional schools have been able to determine their own destinies and incorporate subject fields and disciplines into their curricula as they think best.

Professional schools in the health and hospital administration fields have frequently been submerged in a medical school environment. It is not unusual to find a health school functioning as a small unit of a medical school enterprise and having to clear its budget and curriculum through a maze of medical school committees and deans. A comparable situation exists with management programs in engineering, agriculture, pharmacy, nursing, and education schools. In each of these cases, the school hierarchy tends to be dominated by the academic disciplines. The professional discipline of management and organization tends to be crowded out and there is little concern and an inadequate allocation of resources to programs to train managers. The result is seen in health schools that function at the fourth level down within a medical school, in educational administration programs that have little visibility or prestige within a school of educaton, and a meager, single course in the techniques of management in a large school of engineering.

Experience would seem to indicate that for best results schools of administration, in whatever field, need to have considerable autonomy and independence from other schools and disciplines. This would seem to be one of the preconditions for a profession to come into its own in the management field. In the development of a professional school of health administration, it is essential that the dean or head of the school have status comparable with the other deans in professional management schools of the university.

Focus of the School is the Enlarged Role of the Manager

The education of the health administrator must be focused on a new role, an enlarged function, and a broader set of responsibilities for the manager. Some of the present practitioners will move through this present era and emerge as successful role models and will perform beyond all expectations. Others will move aside to be satisfied with positions of a fairly routine and mechanical nature. The professional schools of health management will turn out younger men and women and will provide refresher programs for practitioners now in the field. Regardless of how the professional school impinges on the life of the young graduate student or the seasoned practitioner, the school will project and seek to reinforce a new function and purpose for the health administrator.

Some of the present schools of health management undoubtedly can shift their interest and resources in new directions to serve the emerging needs of health institutions and the broader community interests. However, several entirely new schools probably should be established and identified as new demonstration models. Considerable experimentation and novel approaches could be tried under controlled conditions in these latter schools. In any event, the issue of how to manage and provide visibility for the professional schools needs to be squarely faced. It is essential that the school have visibility and freedom to develop its own interests and liaisons within the university and within the region being served. Health management deserves to be seen now on a par with industrial and business management and public administration and to develop its own future accordingly. No one discipline or professional subject field should dominate the new school of health management.

Models Will be Different

Different educational models or approaches will be appropriate for different universities and settings. The history, resources, relationships, leadership interests, needs, and make-up of the region itself should be taken into consideration in designing educational programs for health managers. The model sketched out below is in keeping with developments in the Kansas City region, an area of approximately two million population. I draw heavily upon some of the experience we have had to date, especially with our so-called open medical school and with our health sciences programs at the University of Missouri-Kansas City. I also want to acknowledge the contribution of Edgar H. Schien's ideas set out in his exceptionally fine book, *Professional Education—Some New Directions,* a publication of the Carnegie Commission on Higher Education of 1972. In his book, Professor Schein of MIT has summarized and set forth a refreshing and practical framework that deserves the attention of all professional schools of every kind, whether management, engineering, or health sciences.

I sketch out below an approach that I feel would be applicable to the master's degree levels (Master in Health Management) and a professional doctorate (Doctor of Health Management) and that would have application to continuing education efforts as well. There is nothing particularly original about any of the proposals and I am indebted especially to E. Grey Dimond, Provost for the Health Sciences at the University of Missouri-Kansas City, and to Edgar H. Schein of MIT.

The Open School of Health Management

This proposal for a school of health management begins with the concept of the open school, where the environment or region becomes the school itself. Heavy reliance is made upon the resources of the region for faculty and clinical material. The community or region becomes the classroom. One begins by visualizing the ideal, most complete school of health management conceivable, and then searches out within the community the elements and components that would comprise this ideal model.

Hospitals, health care centers, clinics, county-medical societies, Blue Cross, Blue Shield organizations, HEW offices, and many others, are fair game for direct involvement in the open school. All represent potential teaching-learning resources to the school. The professional men and women in these organizations are the potential teachers. An ideal curriculum is fashioned and then matched with what is available in the community and within the university. There is never a perfect fit, but over time the fit improves.

Learning modules are developed, some of one hour in duration and others extending for several weeks or months. The modules are built around desired subject fields, technical topics, skilled areas, workshop exposures, and so forth. Teaching time is purchased from local and visiting resource persons with whatever funds are available to the school. Each student or enrollee can plan his own program and his own track. Some modules may have prerequisites and some may have none at all. Enrollees enter and move through the educational system and participate in the modular settings at their own pace.

Within the school, there is an individualized program for the very young student and there are various educational "packages" for the seasoned practitioner with many years of experience. All are welcome, because there is an appropriate track for all. It is truly a lifetime learning environment.

Within the school, the traditional, campus-based academic programs and lock-step course systems are eliminated or considerably modified. Administrators, trustees, high level technicians, physicians, other medical care professionals, and young graduate students all find an appropriate and useful experience in this setting.

Each module is carefully planned, monitored and evaluated, and is modified as needed by the professional school. Each module is supervised or "taught" by a person or persons competent to handle the subject matter and to integrate theory, applied theory and real life settings. Theory is no longer taught in isolation. Modules themselves would be designed by a team or teams comprised of a management science faculty member, a behavioral scientist, a health practitioner, and perhaps others. Team teaching would be in vogue.

Evaluation methods are established to determine when an individual has demonstrated satisfactory completion or performance for a given module or modular series. Evaluation teams establish methods to assess achievement or capacity levels of individual enrollees in areas of behavioral, cognitive, and analytical skills.

Nature of the Modular Units

Edgar Schein describes well the nature and purpose of the learning modules. Professional education must be organized around a new kind of learning module which:

- Is flexible enough to accommodate students with different learning styles
- Integrates the basic science, applied science, and skill elements to be learned
- Costs less than present comparable educational modules (courses)
- Increases the amount learned by students
- Encourages students to "learn how to learn" so they will be more able to continue their own education following formal schooling. Such modules should also be flexible enough to facilitate the continuing education of alumni of the school at varying periods following graduation and as career switches may be desired.

Real Life Components of the Educational Program

The program described above depends heavily upon cooperation from the health community. The professional school will need to be adept in handling relations with the various partners involved in the total educational undertaking. Some aspects of the health community will be better prepared to work with the professional school than others. Some hospitals and organizations will have ready-made programs in which the school participants can be involved. There will be numerous individuals quite prepared and well qualified to develop modules and to handle the teaching assignments.

However, it will be no easy task to organize the professional school in the health community in a fashion that is satisfactory for professional education purposes. The coordination of modules, real life workshop experiences, and individual student programs will require months if not several years.

Some of the support facilities and program requirements that will be needed by the school include the following:

1. The school will need access to local institutions to serve as demonstration sites for two or more systems of comprehensive health care delivery. The demonstration sites should reflect all or most aspects of primary care medicines, industrial medicine, community health care, home health care, long-term care, nursing home care, rural health care delivery, ghetto programs, etc. The principles of continuity, comprehensiveness and quality should be evident in ongoing programs. These demonstration sites will be major reference points for students and program participants throughout their involvement with the school.

2. The school and its entire program should be affiliated with a university health sciences center, or as a minimum, with a medical center which has education as one of its major concerns.

3. The demonstration sites for medical and health care should have in place or in a planning stage such important systems and methods as the POMR, patient care audits, team care, use of physician's assistants, PSRO's, etc.

4. The participants in the educational programs should have relatively free and random access to every part of the community laboratory. There should be no artificial or unnecessary restraints placed on the students and other enrollees when they are participating in a given module.

5. An efficient data system should be associated with all ongoing health care systems to reflect cost, manpower allocations and performance, patient flows, etc. It is essential that students and program participants get hands on experience with quantitative measurement systems.

6. The school should foster a continuous project of research into major policy issues affecting the health community. The design of adequate health care delivery systems for ghettoes, small communes, and rural areas should be a prime concern. Projects should involve students, faculty, visiting practitioners and community organizations.

7. The education of administrators should be integrated to the greatest extent possible with other health professionals (medical students, medical practitioners, nurses, public health professionals). A major objective of the school of health management should be to reunite in a practical setting the disparate training programs for different kinds of key professionals in the health field. This is especially true of the training programs for these different professionals relating to organization, management and health care delivery.

8. The school should encourage the creation and use of consulting teams comprised of faculty, students, visiting practitioners and others in actual project work in the community. Such projects will provide a major source of case studies and research findings.

9. There is a great value in having at all times a number of practitioners enrolled in the educational programs of the school for periods of three to six months. These programs would provide a sabbatical leave, refresher experience for seasoned administrators.

10. Epidemiology should be taught in a community workshop setting where theory, applied theory and real life activities could be correlated. It would be important for the program participants to view the relationship of health status to housing conditions, employment level, education, diets, income, etc. It perhaps makes little sense to teach epidemiology as an isolated classroom subject.

11. There would be considerable value in creating a community health resource center manned by students and interdisciplinary professional persons. The center might accommodate a range of skilled persons in law, medicine, economics, and health planning to work on major policy and organizational issues in the community. The center would also include the technical consulting arm of the professional school. The consulting unit would concern itself with the more routine organizational and systems needs of health institutions and agencies. It could be anticipated that the community would draw heavily upon the resources center for research into policy issues as well as providing assistance for more technical and routine internal matters within agencies.

12. Special workshops should be offered the year round for health practitioners in the region to acquaint them with new developments in management science, policy analysis, behavioral science applications and other important fields.

13. The school of health management should be closely allied with a clinical management training program for physicians and medical care personnel. There are few programs in the United States which attempt to teach clinical management skills to physicians and other medical care professionals. Many medical centers have the basic clinical materials and organizational systems for such an educational program, but they lack staff and faculty who can handle the management and organization's teaching responsibilities. A soundly conceived clinical management training program for physicians would require a close working partnership between the professional school of health management and the medical school. There is no question that the nation will need more physicians who possess clinical management skills if we are to have efficiently run HMO's, group practice organizations, and make more efficient use of the scarce manpower of our health system.

It would be expecting too much for a school of health management to meet all of these requirements overnight. However, there is no reason to feel that the targets and resources cannot be obtained over a period of time. The main thing is for the school of health management to have a plan and to develop support from the community and from funding sources to make the plan a reality.

Substantive Content of the Educational Program

It is fully anticipated that the educational program would contain at all times adequate substantive content which is provided in many forms such as: full time faculty, adjunct faculty, visiting scholars, audio-visual materials, publications, site visits, work projects, consulting tasks, and job assignments. Much of the course content in an educational program is passed on from student to student. As already indicated, each learning module of the school would seek to incorporate and integrate basic theory, applied theory and a practical workshop. In view of the wide range of learning resources available to teachers and students, there is no reason this cannot be achieved by the school and its affiliates.

The substantive content of the school would cover a wide range of subjects which are basic to the education of a health manager: quantitative measures, health statistics, epidemiology, computer science application, systems analysis, evaluation methods, policy and program development, health law, medical economics, diagnosis of complex systems, planning and managing of change projects, management of task teams, applied behavioral science, and so forth.

It is not possible or practical for a student to cover all of these subjects in a one or two year educational program. Only when an education is a lifetime process can any one practitioner begin to absorb and become skilled in the use of knowledge derived from these various subject fields.

Grouping of Modular Units

If it were felt desirable to categorize or group the various learning modules, there might be some value in developing two major clusters. All of the learning modules of the school might be divided under the following two headings:

- Systems and Medical Care
- Health Policy Analysis and Development

All of the modules would fit in under one of these headings or the other. Subgroupings might be thought of easily within the two major fields.

Additional Features of the School

It would be important for the school to establish a definite policy regarding the recruitment of minority students and enrollees from rural areas. Participants enrolled in the school also should include experienced pro's. There should be a mid-career program for persons currently in the health field as well as for those who are entering the field for the first time.

The school would draw heavily upon persons in the community that could serve as part-time or adjunct faculty. The ratio of adjunct faculty to full time faculty should be in the area of four to one. That is, for each full time faculty member, there should be at least three or four part-time or adjunct faculty members. All persons who serve on the teaching staff, whether full-time or part-time, would have a vote in the policy-making councils of the school. Students also would be represented on all policy and decision-making councils of the school.

Full-time and adjunct faculty, students, and area practitioners all would have voting rights in the governance and administration of the school. Governing and policy councils would make decisions about recruitments, programs design, evaluation methods and selection of faculty.

Peer Relationships within the Educational Environment

Within the school of management, relationships of graduate students, program enrollees, faculty members, senior practitioners, and others take on a whole new meaning. There is some necessary division of responsibilities and separation of roles within the school, but there is a feeling of a common objective for all. Work and study are combined. The curriculum and the learning modules are frequently project centers, where all take an interest in the outcome of the project. As Schein notes, "It is out of such experiences that participants not only learn some of the professional skills, but also gain some self insight, some sense of the value and norms associated with professional roles, and some sense of the difficulties of relating to complex client systems."[12]

Support for the Educational Program

The new and enlarged role for the health manager will gain support as managers perform effectively. There is every reason to anticipate that the administrator will produce and be effective as has been the case in other enterprises in our society. The new role of the manager will win support as the manager performs effectively in institutions and agencies in the community.

The new educational programs of the school of health management must draw on and touch the existing practitioners who have potential for performing an expanded range of functions. The school must attract the young graduate students who will emerge in later years as the new administrator prototype in the health field.

Assume for a moment that there are 20,000 health care managers in the field today who carry heavy or fairly complex responsibility. Let's assume that we have a goal of identifying ten percent or 2,000 of these who are useful role models for the future. Next, assume that there are 50 schools of health management with 15 to 20 management students enrolled. This is a total of 1,000 graduate students per year. Begin to work with these numbers and one senses that by 1980–1985, immense changes in the character of the health administrator's role and image could be fashioned.

HEALTH ADMINISTRATORS WILL HOLD POSITIONS OF RESPONSIBILITY

Where would we expect to find graduates of these new programs five to ten years after graduation? Where would we find the seasoned practitioners who serve as role models and who are closely associated with the new programs in health management?

We can anticipate that the health manager will hold major positions of managerial and staff responsibility with federal agencies, research and consulting firms, congressional and state legislative staff committees, and intermediate positions throughout the health sector. Combined, these individuals will represent a major communications network in itself and will have a major impact on health policy-makers throughout the nation.

Financial Support Will be Needed

Existing and new schools of health management will require considerable financial support from foundations and government in order to launch expanded programs in health administration during the next several years. Funds will be needed for such purposes:

- To finance the purchase of teaching time from adjunct faculty
- To retain faculty and staff members to work directly with and supervise students as they work in the community laboratory setting, and to negotiate work projects on behalf of the students
- To provide audio-visual equipment, supplies, and other materials for student use in recording their experiences and project activities
- To help retain additional faculty members in specialty subject fields with emphasis upon an individual's ability to teach in a practical workshop environment
- To retain consultants in the behavioral science fields and other areas to help design and evaluate the learning modules
- To support the creation, development, and staffing of the community health resource center. This might require three to four full-time equivalent staff positions.

Support from Other Health Care Professionals

There will not be any great surge of support for the new health administrator at first. This makes it all the more imperative that foundation support and encouragement be given to the professional schools that wish to embark on an expanded and new kind of educational format.

It is essential that the programs be continually evaluated and that the end product—namely, the student or enrolled practitioner—be kept in close range during the evaluation process. The educational programs, recruitment process, government funding policies, etc. can be adjusted accordingly.

Respect and support will come from physicians, consumers, community leaders, government administrators, insurance industry executives and others as the new educational programs prove themselves. Ultimately, of course, the proof of the programs will be based on the performance of the administrators themselves.

Nature of the End Product — Health Systems Improvement

We are optimistic that the health manager and graduate of the professional school will prove themselves in a short period of time. The health manager will be used in the community and within his institution as an essential resource for a variety of reasons.

He will be a useful individual because of his trained awareness of human needs. He will be useful in negotiating and planning interrelated programs between institutions. He will possess skills in utilizing people in small group settings. He will be alert to changing needs and trends in social services fields and he will be useful in interpreting the significance of the trends to the trustees and to the community. His systems knowledge and understanding of quantitative methods will be used daily in institutional problem solving. He will be skilled in the use of temporary organizations, and how to involve multiprofessional teams effectively in work settings. Government representatives will call upon him to help to devise better administrative systems and to develop more rational public policy in the health field.

The new role of the health manager will take him out into the community much more than at present. He will be more community oriented and less institutionally oriented. Yet, he will be effective in both environments. He will have the respect of the professional and medical health care personnel because of his ability to create and utilize task and special project groups in improving critically needed systems in the institution. He will be able to teach people who work with him various leadership techniques and approaches. He will be sensitive to other institutional heads and able to relate well and negotiate effectively with them in creating joint systems.

In his enlarged role, the health manager will be involved with other community leaders in designing and evaluating new health care programs and systems that affect the entire community. He will help to establish and manage HMO's, PSRO's, health care foundations, emergency medical services systems, and related endeavors.

The health administrator will know how to use electronic equipment, statistics and quantitative methods which provide the means for evaluating performance and outcome. He will persevere in the use of the data resulting from evaluation systems, even to the point of eliminating unnecessary services and activities.

But the administrator must never lose sight of the purpose and goals of all this quantitative and sophisticated gadgetry. It exists and his career exists only to serve the health needs of individuals, children, women, and men with varying emotional and physical needs.

Conclusion

With health administrators assuming increasingly broader and more important responsibilities in the formulation of policy, the implications are clear. Professional schools of health management must adapt their curricula accordingly. Former HEW Secretary Elliot Richardson has said that, "Our needs for changes in the health care delivery system are great, and schools that train health professionals assume a significant share of the responsibilities for reforming and renovating the system."[13]

Notes

1. E. M. Kennedy. "Senator Kennedy Explains His Health Security Act." *Hospital Progress,* July 1971. Vol. 7, No. 39.
2. W. J. McNerney. "Problems in Financing and Delivery of Care." *Hospital Topics,* July 1971. Vol. 49, No. 34.
3. Kerr L. White. "Life and Death and Medicine." *Scientific American,* September 1973. Vol. 229, No. 3.
4. Cyril O. Schuler. *Hospital Administration,* Winter 1972. Vol. 17, No. 1.
5. Peter F. Drucker. "Managing the Public Service Institution." *Public Interest,* Fall 1973, No. 33. p. 45.
6. Igor H. Ansoff. *Management in Transition, The Conference Board.* New York: The Free Press, 1973.
7. N. J. Stark. "Emerging Role of the Hospital Trustee." Tapes for Trustees, Hospital Trust Fund, 1973.
8. Corine L. Gilb. *Hidden Hierarchies.* New York: Harper & Row, 1966. p. 98.
9. Committee for Economic Development, Research and Policy Committee, *Building a National Health-Care System,* April 1973. p. 61.
10. Herman M. Somers. *Exploring the Future of Health Care.* Syracuse: The Maxwell Summer Lecture Series, 1973. p. 31.
11. Drucker. op. cit. p. 58
12. Edgar H. Schein. *Professional Education: Some New Directions.* New York: McGraw-Hill, 1973. p. 123.
13. Elliot Richardson. Testimony Before the U.S. Senate Labor and Public Welfare Committee, Health Committee. February 22, 1971.

Credentials for Health Administration*

Introduction

The purpose of this paper is to assess and make recommendations regarding credentialing in health administration. Society's need for third party validation of knowledge and competencies of individuals will be given overriding consideration; professional aspirations and goals, often but not always consonant with the commonweal, will be a secondary concern.

The context for the recommendations will be the general meaning, purposes, and uses of credentials in American society. Existing credentialing mechanisms for health administration will be considered. An attempt will be made to match recommendations with the perceived development of health administration as a profession as well as its discernible evolutionary trends.

This paper is by design advocatory with the hope that it will stimulate constructive discussion and debate. Also by design, the author commissioned to write the paper is from outside the academic and practitioner spheres of health administration.

Finally, the emphasis of the paper will be on the usefulness of credentials in a complex and highly technological society. It will, nonetheless, take cognizance of the legions of well documented works on the evils and abuses associated with the maze of credentials in American society. The recommendations will attempt not to fall prey to or create situations where credentialing in health administration will serve the profession to the detriment of the social good.

Credentials and Their Uses in Society

Credentialing in health administration must be considered in the context of the general meaning, purposes, and uses of credentials in

---

* by Jerry W. Miller.

society. Types of credentials and the sources from which they emanate are so varied that a general classification and brief review of their place in the social order will be helpful.

Three general types of credentials are awarded by three general types of authorities:

1. *Degrees, diplomas, and certificates awarded by educational institutions and agencies for successful completion of a specific program of study.* Each educational credential has its own specific meaning, and its meaning and marketplace worth varies with the reputation and quality of the awarding institution. Institutional and/or specialized accreditation, or the lack thereof, are important variables which have a bearing on a credential's value. The credential may qualify the holder for other types of mandatory credentials issued by the government. Or, occupational and professional groups may award the holder certain preferential status. Educational credentials are widely used by business, government, and industry as evidence of desirable employee qualifications.[1] Educational credentials also have a bearing on social status.

2. *Documents of certification, licensure, or registration issued by government to those meeting specific requisites.* These certificates are evidence of the state's permission to engage in a specified activity or to perform a specified act. The agency giving the permission most often has dual authority to prohibit the uncertified from engaging in the specified activity or performing the specified act. Through licensure, the state provides status and recognition to a body of specialized qualifications.

3. *Documents of certification or registration awarded by occupational or professional organizations attesting that the holder meets certain requisites or professional standards.* Holders of such credentials may gain substantial monetary or professional advantage in employment opportunities or in dealing with clients and normally will be afforded greater prestige and deference in professional affairs. Through this process, the profession exercises its self-determined right to regulate and afford recognition to those holding a body of specialized qualifications.

Credentialing involves three parties: (1) the authority issuing the credential, (2) the individual issued the credential, and (3) individuals, groups, or agencies which benefit by or utilize the judgments of the credentialing authority. It involves four principal steps: (1) definition of the attitudes, competencies, knowledge, or skills to be certified, (2) identification of the requisites necessary to qualify for the credential, (3) measurement of individuals to determine whether they meet the requisites, and (4) issuance of a certificate to witness the individual's possession of the requisites. Increasingly, credentialing may involve an important fifth step, that of periodic recertification that the holder continues to possess the requisites for the credentials or has achieved new ones made necessary by advances in the field.

The need for esoteric competencies and knowledge in society gave rise to credentialing as a socially useful concept. Credentialing had its genesis, presumably, through the informal process of a craftsman, trademan, or even a hunter building a reputation in a limited geographical area. As society has grown more complex and science and technology have advanced, credentialing has progressed through the apprentice and guild systems, to degrees and other awards conferred by educational institutions, to credentials awarded by professional associations, to mandatory licensure by government for certain occupations and activities. All of these forms of credentialing are still present in society; moreover, they are expanding and their continued growth is likely to keep pace with society's needs for esoteric services.

Early in the evolution of credentialing, the formal procedure of measuring or making judgments about the qualifications of individuals was instituted. The procedure quickly resulted in the award of a document (credential) attesting that its holder possessed the prescribed qualifications.

Today, the need for some third party validation of occupational or professional qualities is generally accepted as being essential for the effective functioning of society. Most people accept, for example, the need for licensing and other credentials for those who practice medicine, dentistry, and for those who embalm, drive automobiles, and fly airplanes. Moreover, most people would also accept the proposition that all these attitudes, for the good of society, require competencies, knowledge, and skills.

Special note should be made of what a credential certifies: a valid credential means the issuing source has evidence of the holder's qualifications which entitle him to authority and confidence within the area certified. It does not guarantee or assure, however, an adequate performance in every given situation. But the more valid the credential, the more reliable is the performance of the holder, and the more confidence society can have that it will receive adequate services or performances from the credentialed.

The fact that the most numerously and validly credentialed professional commits on occasion a gross error is to be expected. Credentialing is socially useful only because it has a demonstrated capacity to reduce the frequency of such errors. Expectations that credentialing can eliminate error from professional judgments and acts stem from the fact that society expects more than the state of the art of evaluation of the human endeavor can yet deliver. Critics of credentialing rarely acknowledge the immense difficulty of defining the necessary requisites and then determining valid and reliable means of measuring them.

The above is not intended to deny the validiy of much of the criticism directed at credentialing in the United States. The system, heavily dependent on professional subjective judgment and expertise, is pregnant with potential for abuse, error, and social mismanagement and is therefore appropriately suspect. Society must necessarily remain vigilant to these conditions while continuing to recognize its dependence upon credentialing.

Accepting the proposition that at least some credentialing is useful leads to two important questions: (1) What sorts of attitudes, competencies, knowledge, and skills can be validly, reliably, and usefully credentialed? (2) When is it in the interest of society to credential? There are no universally accepted or specific answers to these questions, but some points of information and principles can be identified to guide the considerations.

Society has for hundreds of years identified the parameters of bodies of attitudes, competencies, knowledge, and skills which can be defined, communicated, learned, and believed to be generally essential to an acceptable level of performance of certain acts or services. A specific body of such qualities tends to achieve and maintain a professional or occupational identity even though, the qualities are, ideally, always in a dynamic state. Over an extended period, the dynamism and growth of the necessary requisites may result in the further identification of specialties within a generic classification, such as has happened in medicine, for example. Amidst contending forces and interests, through various means, and usually over considerable periods of time, society has been reasonably efficient in defining and identifying various occupations and professions. Credentialing in its various forms usually emerges simultaneously with the definition and identification. The specific meaning of the resulting credential(s) tends to correlate with the specificity of the definitions and identification.

For illustrative purposes, consider two extremes on the credentialing spectrum: (1) the baccalaureate degree in liberal studies; and (2) the state license to practice dentistry. The latter identifies a very specific skill and body of knowledge; it can be specifically related to educational preparation and experiences; it correlates highly with the reliable delivery of competent services; and it is socially desirable to make credentialing of this activity mandatory. The baccalaureate degree in liberal studies, on the other hand, is not nearly so specific. It is usually indicative of the holder's exposure to a wide variety of subjects in the social, physical, and biological sciences and the arts, humanities, and literature. It may indicate some in-depth study in a specific discipline, but it does not mean that the holder is occupationally or professionally competent to practice in a specific area. That should not be interpreted to denigrate the worth of the credentials, however, for it says a great deal about the holder: mastery of a body of knowledge; the ability to comprehend, synthesize, and analyze quantities of information; the tenacity and drive to accomplish a difficult task and to achieve a personal goal; probability of sensitivity to social issues and problems; and very important to some third parties in the credentialing process, the ability and willingness to learn and master new situations. It is a desired credential but not mandatory in many situations. Between these two extreme of dentistry and liberal studies, there are hundreds of credentials with varying degrees of specificity in meaning.

There appear to be some general principles which speak to the above examples and to the two questions about credentialing. The following are suggested:

1. Credentialing should seek to minimize the risks to the health and safety of the public and individuals by identifying the competent and qualified.

2. Credentialing which recognizes and encourages pride in accomplishment and the mastery of knowledge and skills is in the public interest, because it contributes to the advancement of society and the improvement of the human condition.

3. Mandatory credentialing should be exercised only where there is a demonstrable relationship to the health, safety, and protection of the public.

4. Credentialing intimately related to the health and safety of the public and individuals should periodically require proof that the credentialed still possess the necessary requisites and have kept pace with advances in the field.

5. Credentialing is substantially involved with the system of economic, professional, and social rewards in society. Therefore, it is incumbent upon the system to provide alternate ways of recognizing

attitudes, competencies, knowledge, and skills regardless of how or where they were achieved. To do less is to unjustly discriminate.

6. Credentialing activities of agencies and institutions, whether they are governmentally or publicly controlled, or sponsored by occupational and professional organizations, substantially intersect with the public interest. Their policy-making and governing boards, therefore, should be representative of broad social interests and not confined to a single occupation or profession.

It is within the above context of meanings, purposes, uses, and principles that answers to questions about credentialing in health care administration must be considered.

Health Care Administration as a Profession

Charles J. Austin makes a compelling case (1) that health administration is unique, both as a specialty field of administration and as a function within the health and medical care industry; (2) that health administration must be viewed theoretically in a systems context but also must be looked at as an emerging profession that is taking on the attributes as well as the self-limiting features of professionalism; and (3) that health administration as an area of practice has the potential for steering the larger health and medical care industry into patterns of responsiveness, responsibility, and reconciliation.[2]

Austin acknowledges that health administration has commonalities with other kinds of administration. But he argues forcibly that it has substantial unique characteristics deriving from the idiosyncracies of the health service industry. He makes these important points: (1) the services of the health and medical care industry must be highly individualized; (2) the health and medical care industry is the most highly professionalized and credentialed in society; and (3) the health and medical care system in the United States is extremely complex, involving an intricate network of professional and administrative relationships unrivaled by most other industries. Moreover, he takes a socially attractive judgmental position that health administration should become the locus in the health and medical care industry for providing accountability to its constituencies and society.

Austin also makes the point, however, that health administrators are not the only participants in the process of health administration—they share responsibility with physicians, nurses, other health professionals, politicians, community leaders, and governmental officials. And, health administrators are not in total control of their own activities, let alone all aspects of the larger health and medical care system.

Additionally, health administrators serve in a broad variety of roles and organizational situations, calling for different educational preparation and work experieneces. Austin names four major categories: health care statesmen, organizational executives, middle management personnel, and administrative staff specialists. They administer large hospital complexes, community health centers, medical clinics, long-term care facilities, health maintenance organizations, public health agencies, and nursing homes. In addition, Austin makes this point:

> . . . different kinds of administrators may be required in different phases of the life of an organization or health program. The social entrepreneur needed to plan and develop a new medical center may be quite ineffective as an operational manager at a period of more stability in the activities of this organization.

In addition, many entry level positions in health administration do not yet require specific preparation in the field. Individuals may still become top-level health administrators through on-the-job experience. But there is an apparent growing tendency in the direction of specific educational requirements and preference by employers for those specifically educated in health administration.

As a professional group, health administration is a specialty in transition and evolution. The creation of the Commission on Education for Health Administration is partial acknowledgement of that fact. The rapidly changing patterns of health care delivery—the new structures, relationships, professional identities, and organizations those changes are spawning—are additional proof of the dynamic state of the profession, its pains, opportunities, and social importance.

In advocating a credentialing system for health administration, the broad definition of the profession, its transitory state, and its growing importance to society as an instrumentality which promises greater efficiency, effectiveness, and equity in health care delievery must be considered. Also, so must its legitimate aspirations as a profession as well as its aspiration to share in the economic and social rewards society allows other professions.

For purposes of this paper, Austin's theses and terminology of health administration as a profession are accepted without debate. His analysis has utility because it defines a body of attitudes, competencies, knowledge, and skills which should be associated with the practice of health administration. But the status of health administration as a profession, while interesting, is not the primary reason for credentialing; social usefulness is, or should be. And, as has been shown before, credentialing is socially useful regardless of the professional status of the activity being credentialed.

The status of an occupation as a profession does have some bearing on the arrangements and mechanisms for credentialing, however. The greater the clarity of a group's claim that only its members possess a body of competencies, knowledge, and skills which are essential to society, the more likely it will be granted a high degree of autonomy. With his grant of autonomy comes the right to substantial control of the credentialing process, whether it be state or professionally operated, or involves certification of individuals or accreditation of educational programs. And, the greater the clarity of the claim, the greater the worth of the status conferred.

Existing Credentialing System in Health Administration

Like the profession, the existing credentialing system in health administration is in transition. The granting of specific types of degrees in health administration, the specialized accreditation of schools and departments within colleges and universities awarding these degrees, professional association membership, and state licensure are all on the increase. All are part of the credentialing system. Their value in the marketplace and their worth as reliable indications of the quality of individuals would be difficult to determine and are beyond the scope of this paper. It is useful, nonetheless, to examine the current credentialing scene.

Degrees Awarded by Educational Institutions

Educational institutions award degrees at the associate, baccalaureate, master's and doctoral levels in fields which find their generic home in health administration. These degrees, nearly all awarded by regionally accredited institutions, generally indicate the following about the holder: some mastery of a body of knowledge in general or liberal education; mastery of a body of knowledge relating to health administration; the ability to comprehend, synthesize, and analyze quantities of information; the tenacity and drive to accomplish a difficult task and to achieve a personal goal; and the ability and willingness to master new situations in a reasonable period of time. The presumed value of the degree varies with the individual and the presumed quality of the institution.

Degrees Awarded by Educational Institutions Whose Programs Hold Specialized Accreditation

In health administration, the Accrediting Commission for Graduate Education in Hospital Adminisration accredits programs of study specifically preparing health administrators. The American Public Health Association accredits schools of public health which may also have programs preparing health administrators, and the American Association of Collegiate Schools of Business accredits components of colleges and universities which sometimes have programs of study in health administration.

Specialized accreditation provides special assurance, in addition to regional accreditation, concerning the quality of specific programs of study. It provides a more extensive and intensive evaluation, bringing to bear the viewpoints of both educators and practitioners with regard to the quality and relevancy of educational programs. It speaks to similarity of objectives among educational programs, and—within a reasonable range—to the uniformity of the educational process and comparability of graduates. Holders of degrees validated by specialized accreditation should be expected to possess essentially the same attributes listed for degree holders in general, but there should be less variance in the quality. Additionally, graduates of programs holding specialized accreditation warrant greater confidence and higher expectations of professional performance.

Membership and Other Status in Professional Associations

A number of professional associations serve the field of health administration, including the American College of Hospital Administrators, the American College of Nursing Home Administrators, the Association of Mental Health Administrators, the Medical Group Management Association, the Hospital Financial Management Association, the American Association of Comprehensive Health Planning, the American Public Health Association, and the American Academy of Health Administration. Requirements for the levels of status with these associations are varied. Professional association membership is mentioned here, because it is assumed to have a positive relationship to the requisite competencies and skills needed in health administration. For illustrative purposes, membership requirements for two of the organizations, the American College of Hospital Administrators

(ACHA) and the American College of Nursing Home Administrators (ACNHA) will be examined in some detail.

Pertinent requirements covering initial admission and advancement categories in ACHA are as follows:

Nomineeship—A baccalaureate degree or a graduate degree from a program accredited by the Accrediting Commission on Graduate Education for Hospital Administration is required. A candidate with a baccalaureate degree must have at least three years of responsible experience in an acceptable situation. Graduate degree holders need only one year of experience. A candidate with a baccalaureate degree must be an administrator, assistant administrator, or administrative assistant or hold an equivalent position. The graduate degree holder must be in a "responsible administrative position" in an acceptable situation.

Membership—Membership may be granted after three years of nominee status if oral and written examinations are passed and a responsible administrative position is maintained. Nominees are required to complete the requirements for membership within five years after admission.

Fellowship—This status may be awarded to a member of at least six years tenure who has satisfactorily completed other requirements which include evidence of service to the hospital field beyond the ordinary demands of the position, including participation in the affairs of the College and other health-field activities, as a professional leader in administration, and a program of continuing education for personal growth and development, and a Fellowship project or a thesis or four case reports.[3]

ACNHA has similar categories of status covering admission and advancement within the organization. Pertinent requirements are as follows:

Nominee—Actively engaged in the practice of nursing home administration, and such other general qualifications as established by the Board of Governors.

Member—Be a nominee in good standing and recommended for advancement by two Fellows; be a licensed nursing home administrator in the jurisdiction in which he practices; have at least two years of experience; and meet other general requirements as established by the Board of Governors.

Fellow—Be a member in good standing for at least two years and be recommended for advancement by three Fellows; must have completed at least four years of training beyond high school, or equivalency at the discretion of the Board of Governors; give evidence of service beyond the ordinary demands of his position and of continued adherence to the criteria for membership.[4]

Licensure—Two states, Alabama and Minnesota, have licensure laws for hospital administrators. A 1968 survey by the American Hospital Association revealed that six other states had regulations affecting registration of hospital administrators, and 11 were planning licensure programs.

State licensure for those administering nursing homes was mandated by the 1967 Social Security Amendments (P.L. 90-248) if states participating in the Medicaid program wished to continue to receive federal funds. This federal requirement apparently came as a result of the recognition of the low level of care provided by some nursing homes under existing state regulations. Important to the consideration of credentialing in health administration, it also recognized the a priori assumption that the nursing home administrator is the key to the level of care provided in that particular type of health care institution. Moreover, it also recognized that no other credentialing mechanism was in place which could provide assurances about minimum threshold competencies for the nursing home administrator.

Other types of licensure or state regulation—to the extent that they exist—do not appear to be major factors in the credentialing of health administrators.

Objectives for Credentialing in Health Administration

The following objectives for credentialing in health administration are postulated:

1. Credentialing in health administration should seek to provide assurances regarding minimally acceptable competencies for those serving as the chief administrators of health agencies and organizations, particularly where there is limited opportunity for day-to-day interaction and sharing of responsibility with other health professionals.

2. Credentialing in health administration should recognize and encourage sound educational preparation and achievement for all entry levels and specialties in health administration.

3. Credentialing in health administration should encourage and reward, if not require, continuing education as a means of keeping administrators current with advances in the field.

4. Credentialing in health administration should encourage and promote advanced study beyond the educational level needed for entry into the field and provide incentives for practitioners without acceptable competencies and skills to engage in formal educational programs.

5. Credentialing in health administration should provide means whereby relevant attitudes, competencies, knowledge, and skills held by the currently uncredentialed can be given equitable recognition.

Proposals for Credentialing in Health Administration

In keeping with the objectives postulated for credentialing in health administration, the following proposals speak primarily to the need for assuring threshold or entry level competencies, continuing education, advanced study, and equitable recognition of requisites regardless of where and how these were achieved. The proposals also seek to achieve some balance of power among credentialing agencies.

EDUCATIONAL PREPARATION

The transitory state of the health administration profession, the rapidly evolving and diverse situations and relationships among which it is expected to practice, and its ill-defined nature and varying competency levels indicate a need for generalized types of credentials for entry level purposes at this point in the development of the profession.

Educational credentials meet this requirement and have one other distinct advantage: they are less likely to retard desirable evolution of the profession. Institutions of higher education, which will be preparing the bulk of health administrators in the future, are under fewer restraints in responding to manpower needs than are other credentialing agencies—state licensure boards and professional and occupational certifying groups. Being controlled primarily or exclusively by the profession, these agencies understandably are inclined to protect their own professional and economic interests and consequently often thwart marketplace demands.

It should be noted, however, that institutions appear to be less than responsive to marketplace manpower needs at two stages of development of professions or occupations: (1) very early in the development; and (2) after several years of evolution when the occupational or professional identity has become solidified. Health administration falls between those two extremes. Institutions of higher education by the hundreds have discovered health administration as a current manpower need and a major field of preparation and have instituted varying types of curricula. Therein lies a blessing but, from the viewpoint of many, also a problem.

Institutions will be producing a wealth of health administrators to meet manpower requirements, but it may not be of the ilk perceived as needed by either the marketplace or the more established components of the profession. Thus, an age-old struggle takes on new vigor in yet another field. There is a need for some standardization of educational programs, on the one hand, and the profession's continued need to develop and evolve, on the other. Other components of the struggle are the desire of the educational institution to be as free as possible of external constraints versus the profession's constant effort to shape and control its own destiny—education being a major tool. Such is the battleground and state of tension for the milieu of specialized accreditation.

Many administrators of institutions and representatives of regional accreditation are prepared to argue—and have for years—that institutional accreditation is sufficient to speak to the quality of all or most programs of study offered by a regionally accredited institution. Representatives of the professions and institutional faculty closely aligned with professional groups are prepared to argue just as forcibly—and have for years—that specialized accreditation is needed to assure educational quality for practice-oriented programs of study. Research supporting either position is virtually nonexistent, but there is the general belief that educational preparation is the single most reliable measure of occupational competence. The quality of the educational preparation is then obviously a factor.

Regardless of the merits of these arguments about institutional and specialized accreditation, at least the limited use of specialized accreditation in higher education is winning the day, and for good and practical reasons. Specialized accreditation with a well developed social and educational conscience has more to offer institutions than passing on the quality of their programs. In a dynamic field such as health administration, it can provide assistance in curriculum design and development; it can provide institutions wth consultative services and a critical mass of expertise; and it can help institutions strike a balance between the needs of professional practice and pure educational considerations.

Moreover, specialized accreditation has value to employers and others who have a need for third party validation of the qualifications of individuals. Mechanisms will evolve to meet these credentialing needs if educational institutions do not. Credentialing through educational preparation at this point in the development of the profession, further validated by specialized accreditation, will tend to keep other more restrictive credentialing from evolving.

Additionally, degree programs at the associate, baccalaureate, and graduate levels probably can be reasonably matched with the threshold and entry level competency requirements of the marketplace. At the same time, this type of credentialing will tend to promote and encourage advanced study, thereby creating avenues for upward and geographic mobility in the profession which can be based on a combination of administrative experience and formal degree programs. Advanced study will also enhance the field's scholarly development.

The graduate hospital administration component of health administration has a well-established and functionally effective system of specialized accreditation for programs of study preparing hospital administrators. Membership of this agency, already representative of diverse interests in the profession, could be expanded to cover other areas and levels of educational preparation for health administration. Other agencies, if they were to be created, would have to go through long periods of development and the pangs of being officially and unofficially recognized as legitimate and authoritative arbiters of quality.

Great care should be exercised in expanding specialized accreditation for health administration because of the nature of the process. Specialized accreditation loses its reason for being as its continuum approaches that of institutional accreditation. It is most rational, acceptable, and effective when its claim to expertise is clear, in least dispute, and when it can concentrate on a well-defined area.

Education preparing administrators to manage clinics, health maintenance organizations, hospitals, long-term care facilities, and nursing homes which provide direct patient care is a reasonably esoteric area, only mildly disputed by those who argue for a generic educational approach for the training of all types of administrators. Beyond that fairly clear claim, however, health administration spills over into contested territory. Health care planning and the administration of health agencies not involved in the direct delivery of patient care are areas of expertise and intense interest on the part of political and social scientists, environmental and sanitation engineers, public administrators, and planners of various designations, including the generic type. Encompassing such disputed areas in a program of specialized accreditation at this point in the development of health administration would be counter-productive. Moreover, it could circumscribe a field of endeavor which may have more affinity with community, environmental, and public health.

Recommendation: (1) That the Accrediting Commission on Graduate Education for Hospital Administration be reorganized to accredit all levels and programs of study preparing individuals to administer organizations involved in the direct delivery of patient care, (2) that

specialized accreditation be the principal means of meeting the needs of threshold and entry level credentialing for this area of health administration, and (3) that programs of study preparing other types of health administrators be subjected only to institutional accreditation pending further development of the profession.

LICENSURE

Conditions in the field appear to warrant a credential which can speak to threshold requisites for administering certain types of health care delivery institutions. The state licensure laws enacted to meet the requirements of the 1967 Social Security Amendments are an attempt to assure the competency of individuals administering nursing homes.

The federal legislation was enacted because sufficient numbers of individuals holding educational credentials attesting to threshold requisites were not available and unlikely to be for a considerable period of time. The more encompassing responsibility required of the health administrator in this particular type of health care institution was also a factor. The influence of the day-to-day contact and shared responsibility for the delivery of services with other highly credentialed professionals in the health fields, such as is the case with the hospital administrator, is much less for this type of administrator. Other conditions, such as private ownership, also bear on the need for such threshold credentialing.

It is interesting to note that as state agencies and professional groups grapple with the problems of implementing licensure laws for nursing home administrators, they turn virtually automatically to formal educational preparation as a principal screening device, although testing is being used.

Licensure laws, once enacted, are sometimes amended but rarely abolished. Ideally, at some point in the future, licensure will become primarily a function of education. Ideally, also, other licensure laws will not be enacted for health care administrators, relying instead on other types of credentials.

Recommendation: (1) That licensure for nursing home administrators move rapidly toward educational requisites, and, (2) that third party validation requirements for other types of administrators, who share responsibilities with governing boards and other health professionals, be met by other credentials.

Continuing Education

In a rapidly developing specialty, credentials quickly become dated and provide little assurance that the holder has kept up with advances in the field. Health administration credentialing appears to qualify as a field needing required continuing education.

This need presents a unique opportunity for professional associations to make membership in their organizations a more meaningful credential. It also presents the organizations with opportunities to assist the health administration profession in pursuing specialized competencies and further professional development, building on study in formal degree programs at both the undergraduate and graduate levels. It also presents each of the associations with the opportunity to service and focus on a membership with homogeneous interests and needs.

Continuing education will be addressed in another Commission paper, but some points should be noted here. Continuing education for the purposes of keeping credentials current requires a different structure and measurement of student achievement than other types of organized noncredit, avocational types of educational programs which also carry the designation. It also is different from the set of academic experiences required for degree programs. It requires some validation that the providing institution or agency is qualified to offer the programs; it also requires a system of student record keeping which meshes with the credentialing system it updates.

Meeting the continuing education needs of the field will require substantial cooperation among professional associations and educational institutions.

Recommendation: (1) That professional associations in health administration adopt appropriate educational requirements as a base criterion for membership, (2) that the associations adopt appropriate continuing education requirements for maintaining membership and as evidence of continuing occupational competency, and (3) that a formal or informal council of health administration professional associations and associations of institutions offering education for health administration be formed to coordinate and consider continued education needs of the profession.

Under this sort of arrangement, professional associations will be serving meaningful public functions closely akin to the quasi-governmental functions now served by nongovernmental accrediting agencies. It is therefore proposed that this be appropriately recognized in the organization of the associations.

Recommendation: That members of professional association bodies which make and administer policy with regard to initial and continued membership requirements contain the educational and practice interests of the profession and individuals who are not educators or practitioners in health administration.

External Degrees Opportunities

The foregoing recommendations rely heavily upon education as the principal means of providing assurances about the attitudes, competencies, knowledge, and skills of health administrators. The recommendations could be subject to considerable criticism on that point alone if it is assumed that the education proposed is the traditional, resident type of formal study. It is not.

Society and educators are coming to recognize that education occurs in many ways and in many settings. Some of education is the formally structured, supervised educational experience. Education, as the Commission on Non-Traditional Study pointed out, also takes place through nonrequired reading, learning on-the-job, and a host of other informal educational experiences. The former results usually, upon the successful completion of a prescribed program of study, in the award of an educational credential. Until recently, the latter went uncredentialed and often unrewarded, resulting in barriers for the individual seeking economic and professional opportunities.

Two principal types of degree programs, generically called external degrees, but perhaps more usefully labeled nonresident, have emerged in the United States: (1) the validating external degree, and (2) the external degree which can be earned through nonresident study.

External or nonresident degrees for health administration, providing both the validating and nonresident study components, should be instituted for two principal reasons: (1) social justice demands that the many noncertified practitioners in health administration, who hold the requisite qualifications, be provided with the opportunity to become credentialed and participate in the economic, professional, and social opportunities afforded those who have been credentialed through traditional means, and (2) upgrading of the practice of health administration could be substantially improved by providing current practitioners with opportunities to study through nonresident degree programs.

The Association of University Programs in Health Administration has already taken steps to institute nonresident educational programs for health administration. Such efforts should be applauded and supported.

Recommendation: (1) That the Association of University Programs in Health Administration continue to serve as the catalytic agent to bring about institutional or consortium-based external degree programs, and (2) that steps be taken to assure that these are programs of high quality in order to enhance their acceptance by employers, licensure agencies, and professional associations on the same basis as traditional credentials.

Creation of a validating model of the external degree for health administration will substantially reduce the socially discriminatory aspects of credentialing. It will provide the opportunity for due recognition of educational achievement and merit.

Interlocking arrangements among credentialing authorities—educational institutions, licensure agencies, and professional associations—also have their discriminatory aspects. Graduation from an educational program holding specialized accreditation is a reasonable means of establishing eligibility for membership in some professional associations. But alternate means should be provided also for those who have graduated from unaccredited programs of study. Alternate means of meeting the educational requirements for licensure should also be provided.

Recommendation: (1) That until validating models of the external degree are available, professional associations and licensure agencies should employ methods such as norm-referenced standardized testing to satisfy educational criteria for those who do not hold a credential or have not graduated from an accredited program, and (2) that if part one of this recommendation is adopted, employers should view membership in a professional association as an adequate alternative to specialized accreditation.

NOTES

1. Throughout this paper the terms "requisites" and "qualifications" are used to refer to a body of attitudes, competencies, knowledge, and skills.
2. Charles J. Austin. "What is Health Administration?" A Working Paper prepared for the Commission on Education for Health Administration, October, 1973.
3. *Directory of the American College of Hospital Administrators, 1972.* Chicago: The College, 1972. p. xviii.
4. *The Bylaws of the American College of Nursing Home Administrators, 1973.* Silver Spring, MD: The College, 1973. pp. 2–3.

Career Mobility and Lifelong Learning in Health Administration*

Introduction

The purpose of this paper is to link the concept of lifelong learning to the development of a new profession by utilizing strategies for continuous and continuing education and assessment which might affect career development, certification, and performance effectiveness. I have chosen to use a *global* perspective rather than a *reductionist* technical approach, since I cannot effectively separate the education of professionals from the process of professionalization.

A Cursory Sociology of Health Administration and Health Administration Education

Everett C. Hughes is quoted by Vollmer and Mills[1] as saying "In my own studies I passed from the false question 'Is this occupation a profession?' to the more fundamental one, 'What are the circumstances in which people in an occupation attempt to turn it into a profession and themselves into professional people?' " In this spirit, I'd like to engage in a cursory examination of health administration as a set of occupational clusters.

ORGANIZATIONS OF THE PROFESSION

The rubric of health administration leads the uninformed observer to believe that there is a single, well organized occupational group which has achieved some level of professionalism and is now striving to continue its development in a more contemporary mode. Further examination leads the observer to note the existence of such professional associations as the American College of Hospital Administrators

---

* by Stephen B. Plumer.

and the American College of Nursing Home Administrators, each with a distinctive history, sense of mission, and a membership with diverse educational and experiential backgrounds. Each of these groups has membership categories, e.g., Fellow, which signifies a level of achievement and professional recognition. There is, however, a licensure procedure for Nursing Home Administrators which operates outside of the definition and control of the ACNHA. In addition, there is a variety of trade associations whose memberships are primarily institutional, e.g., American Hospital Association. There are also associations whose membership is composed of both individuals and organizations, e.g., Association of Mental Health Administrators.

Within each category of association the statement of mission includes a concern with the quality of service to be provided to the consumer and an implicit, linking concern with the quality of educational preparation of the person responsible for administering the delivery of the service.

Within the health administration rubric there is also the Association of University Programs in *Health* Administration (AUPHA) which recently changed its name from the Association of University Programs in *Hospital* Administration. This Association, which is the primary, visible representation of health administration education, is a consortium of approximately 50 percent of the operating programs in the health administration field and has provided leadership in the creation of an accrediting mechanism for such programs. The history of university programs in the field is the history of a diminishing role of practitioners as faculty until, today, the programs are dominated by persons whose careers are rooted in the occupational cluster of a health administration education with what appears to be a commitment to remain in the academic setting.

There is no association of health administration educators. It should be noted that faculty members of various programs do work together on specific tasks under the auspices of AUPHA. They do so, however, as employees of a member program and not as a group of professionals with a distinctive identity. In other contexts, e.g., APHA, these same faculty come together with practitioners on more global issues, and function more as expert professionals than as "program faculty."

The Occupational Settings

As an employe, the health administrator works for a set of organizations which are devoted to the delivery of various professional services. The characteristics of the organizational setting have a significant effect on the health administrator's self-image, definition of client, and concept of the appropriate ways to relate to the client.[2]

The increasing complexity of the health delivery system has created a situation in which the health consumer as client is frequently displaced by organized sets of employes, professional providers, third-party payment agencies, regulatory agencies, and community groups of non-clients representing consumer/client interests.

The variety of competing demands by the nonconsumer creates a goal displacement for the administrator and, therefore, for the institution. Initially, the function of this displacement forces the health administrator to utilize his skills to resolve internal problems, presumably to improve service to clients. The result of this preoccupation with internal problem-solving becomes an end in itself and results in "we're doing the best that we can do under the circumstances," or "the union's lack of concern about patients has made it difficult to...." This phenomenon has impacted on the consumer and aided in the emergence of the new activism demanding greater responsiveness and accountability.

LITERATURE

The literature of the field is dispersed through a variety of journals and in each case acknowledges the increasingly complex organizational settings, the need for improved management skills (financial, personnel, computer applications and systems analysis), and a more thorough grounding in understanding medical-nursing practice. As is the case with most fledgling emerging professions which relate intimately to *the profession* of medicine, there is considerable self-deprecation, preoccupation with status, and efforts to emulate medicine in order to improve self-image and possible job effectiveness. (Could it be that the low esteem of the nursing home administrator is related to the absence of gerontological medicine as a specialty?)

CONTINUING EDUCATION

Continuing education in the field is a euphemism for non-credit and/or certificate programs offered by professional associations, regional centers, and some colleges and universities with health administration programs for purposes of: assisting practitioners to meet licensure requirements; upgrading practitioner on-the-job performance—encouraging peer interaction and self-improvement; providing identification and certification within the professional subgroup. Continuing education seems to have the potential of being a subindustry in the field. For this reason it may be important to understand the economics of the existing continuing education activities as well as the levels of participation by various subgroups compared to the potential participation. The W. K. Kellogg Foundation has been instrumental in developing a broad spectrum of activities in the field and is regarded with respect and mixed affect by both the practitioner and educator. The mixed affect is generated by those who wish that the Foundation would give money and leave intervention and control to the qualified professionals, and those who are thankful for the Foundation's openness and unwillingness to allow premature closure.

The Commission on Education for Health Administration

There is apprehension in the field, at this point, about how the work of the Commission on Education for Health Administration will affect the future policies and practices of the W. K. Kellogg Foundation with regard to its support for health administration. There is also concern about the impact of the Commission on existing power and influence configurations within the field.

Definition of Health Administration

The interim report of the Commission, released August, 1973, defines health administration as "planning, organizing, directing, controlling, coordinating, and evaluating the resources and procedures by which needs and demands for health and medical care and a healthful environment are fulfilled, by the provision of specific services for individual clients, organizations and communities." In addition to this general definition, Commission minutes and staff working papers emphasize the importance of the leadership role of the health administrator as a consumer/client advocate and as a change agent. Emphasis is also placed on the need for health administration to develop an expanded view of professionalism which is both accountable and responsive. There is limited data available from which to examine existing practice and the interventions which would be necessary to assist the health administrator in becoming a client advocate and change agent.

Demographic Data

Although we have access to demographic data about some categories of health administrators linking age, schooling, and years of experience with types of positions held, there is no aggregate data about career patterns and mobility of the practicing administrator, nor is there any data about the socio-economic and personality variables which help us to understand patterns of career choice. The studies currently being conducted by the Commission and the membership data from the professional associations do not take into account the need to understand career patterns from the point of selection, and to relate aspiration to self-perceived success. Another need is to understand enough about the personal characteristics of the practitioner to know whether existing personnel or the new entrants in the field can become effective advocates, change agents, or have the capacity to engage with clients in accountability behaviors which require reciprocity and intensive interpersonal encounters.

Generally speaking, the outside observer is struck by: the clubiness among the health administrator practitioners and educators; the intensity of cults of personality; the evaluation of practicing professionals by personal characteristics and mannerisms on a comparable level with professional concerns; the primitive and awkward politics for control and leadership in the development of professionalism; a disconnectedness with trends in higher education and professional education; a competitiveness between practitioners and educators for control of definitions of professionalism.

It can be concluded that the occupational clusters of health administration and health administration education are healthfully exhibiting behaviors consistent with their stage of development as marginal or emerging professions.

Old and New Professionalism

Schein presents a comprehensive list of criteria which, in global terms, defines a classic profession and which when applied to a specific occupational group can be used to measure the degree of professionalization which it has achieved.[3]

1. The professional, as distinct from the amateur, is engaged in a full-time occupation that comprises his principal source of income.

2. The professional is assumed to have a strong motivation or calling as a basis for his choice of a professional career and is assumed to have a stable lifetime commitment to that career.

3. The professional possesses a specialized body of knowledge and skills that are acquired during a prolonged period of education and training.

4. The professional makes his decisions on behalf of a client in terms of general principles, theories, or propositions, which he applies to the particular case under consideration, i.e., by "universalistic" standards, in terms of Parsons' pattern variables.

5. At the same time, the professional is assumed to have a service orientation, which means that he uses his expertise on behalf of the particular needs of his client. This service implies diagnostic skill, competent application of general knowledge to the special needs of the client, and an absence of self-interest.

6. The professional's service to the client is assumed to be based on the objective needs of the client and independent of the particular sentiments that the professional may have about the client. The professional promises a "detached" diagnosis. The client is expected to be fully frank in revealing potentially unlikeable things about himself; the professional, as his part of the contract, is expected to withhold moral judgment, no matter how he may feel personally about the client's revelation. Thus, the professional relationship rests on a kind of mutual trust between the professional and client.

7. The professional is assumed to know better what is good for the client than the client himself. In other words the professional demands autonomy of judgment of his own performance. Even if the client is not satisfied, the professional will, in principle, permit only his colleagues to judge his performance. Because of this demand for professional autonomy, the client is in a potentially vulnerable position. How does he know whether he has been cheated or harmed? The profession deals with this potential vulnerability by developing strong ethical and professional standards for its members. Such standards may be expressed as codes of conduct and are usually enforced by colleagues through professional associations or through licensing examinations designed and administered by fellow professionals.

8. Professionals form professional associations which define criteria of admission, educational standards, licensing or other formal entry examinations, career lines within the profession, and areas of jurisdiction for the profession. Ultimately, the professional association's function is to protect the autonomy of the profession; it develops reasonably strong forms of self-government by setting rules or standards for the profession.

9. Professionals have great power and status in the area of their expertise, but their knowledge is assumed to be specific. A professional does not have a license to be a "wise man" outside the area defined by his training.

10. Professionals make their service available but ordinarily are not allowed to advertise or to seek out clients. Clients are expected to initiate the contact and then accept the advice and service recommended, without appeal to outside authority.

We need to acknowledge that these criteria, although they number ten, are not etched in stone, nor do they possess divine qualities.

Items 2 and 3 are rooted in the history of a single occupational choice of being normative and a concept of schooling which equates learning with time spent in school. The rapid changes in technology and economics (ask an aeronautical or space engineer) create an environment of career change as do the phenomena of increased leisure time, early retirement and a more accessible educational system. We have learned enough about expectation theory to be suspicious of Item 6, while the emergence of malpractice suits and community interventions create a challenge for Item 7. Despite these limitations, these ten criteria can be modified and applied to an examination of the practice of health administration and its processes of professionalization.

Schein is also helpful in identifying the complexities of an emerging multiple client system in which the organization (worksetting) can be a client in some ways, while within the organization or the society at large, the division of labor produces a set of immediate, intermediate and ultimate clients.

> ... The phenomenon of professional services that are initially commissioned by one client system (the immediate) and are evaluated by an intermediate client system even though they are carried out in behalf of some ultimate use of the products of the service (ultimate client) ..."[4]

> ... The hiring of an architect by a real estate firm to build low-cost housing with the aid of federal funds administered through a local housing authority. The real estate firm is the immediate client, the housing authority is the intermediate client, and the low income tenant is the ultimate client. This example can be further complicated by considering as intermediate clients the local planning authority, which attempts to integrate the housing development aesthetically into some larger plan for the city, and the local city government which considers the tax-base implications of the development. An additional ultimate client is the public at large, which wants a housing development that will not only be aesthetically pleasing but will reduce some social ills of the ghetto.[5]

The complexity of this situation is further illustrated when 'the low income tenant wants inexpensive, flexible housing that will permit the expression of his cultural norms and values; the real estate developer . . . will be guided by efficiency, not by relevance to the cultural values of the tenants; the housing authority wants housing that will fit into its overall master plan of urban development and *its* set of assumptions about the needs of the ghetto dweller. The architect will also be highly responsive to his own assumptions and to the style of his firm . . . Given these forces it is unlikely that the ghetto dwellers' needs and culture will be high on the list of client concerns to be taken into account.[6]

It seems to be true that a new professionalism will result in greater roles for the ultimate clients and that these new roles will be a function of self-protection for the professional (involvement of a patient in a treatment decision about an incurable malignancy), as well as a recognition of the fact that new standards and ethics are necessary to maximize professional effectiveness. In order to progress through the process of professionalization, there is a need to gather data about the multiple client systems which health administrators serve and to clarify the abstractions of advocacy, accountability, and social change in light of these analyses.

Although the need for specific research is of critical importance, there are some steps which might be experimented with now. Professional associations can develop some continuing education activities which bring together clients and professionals around topics of mutual concern. They might also wish to develop liaison with national consumer groups and ultimately may wish to create an auxiliary membership category for persons who are part of their multiple client system. Academic programs may want to build input from clients into both an instructional and action research mode, in order to assist the student to learn to engage in new collaborative behaviors.

These brief "almost suggestions" are presented by way of acknowledging the fact that there is a tendency to protect marginality by creating limited access and "super-professional" window-dressing. It is also acknowledged that professional associations in all fields are the most conservative, since they are often controlled by their older, established members whose careers are rooted in a different era of success definitions. For this reason, I am suggesting that survival can be viewed from an initiatory, positive stance, as well as from a reactive defensive one.

Just a word more about careers and their relation to the process of professionalization. A career is a set of constant adjustments between a person, his/her professional world and the facets of his/her everyday life. "It involves the running of risks, for his career is his ultimate enterprise, his laying of bets on his one and only life."[7] Any changes in circumstances which threaten this basic sense of self and personal investment results in a fear of the unknown future, and a perpetuation of past "successful ways of doing things." Schein hit the nail on the head when he stated, "No matter how much pressure is put on a person or social system to change through disconfirmation and the induction of guilt-anxiety, no change will occur unless the members of the system feel it is safe to give up the old responses and learn something new."[8]

Lifelong Learning, Continuing and Continuous Education

THE TRADITION OF CONTINUING EDUCATION IN HEALTH ADMINISTRATION

One of my intentions in preparing this paper was to report on the state of the art in Continuing Education for Health Administration. Much to my dismay I discovered that there is no central source for the specification, collection and analysis of data about such activities. Impressionistically, I can report that continuing education activities are conducted by some trade associations (e.g., AHA), the professional associations, and a variety of colleges and universities. One-day in-and-out sessions, two-day seminars, one-week workshops, and quarter/semester long activities are included in the variety of offerings. Many programs offered by the college and university set offer certificates for successful completion, some offer college credit and none offer degree programs, although the University of Minnesota has provision for the transfer of credits, at an undergraduate level, with several cooperating colleges and universities in its area.

An examination of program announcements, descriptions and annual reports yields the view that ACHA and ACNHA use very few faculty members as experts/trainers/workshop leaders. For the most part management consultants, other professionals (e.g., lawyers, architects, accountants, systems analysts) and experienced specialized practitioners provide the basic source of expertise. The higher education programs use some faculty (estimated at less than 10 percent in a Commission survey of the graduate programs) and attempt to utilize practicing professionals for their practicality and ability to legitimize the program (being sure that the practitioner does not regard the content as being too abstract).

Although there is an unevenness in what is reported or available, there is no evaluative data or other basis on which to evaluate either quality or effectiveness. On the other hand, the reports of the Hospital Continuing Education Project (HCEP) report data about hospital continuing education in a goal-directed project. The data from some of the centers indicates impact on career mobility, improved performance and sense of personal growth and satisfaction. (See, for example, "Universities, Colleges, and Hospitals: Partners in Continuing Education" published by W. K. Kellogg Foundation updated.)

In a national survey of hospital administrators, Matzick reports a high level of satisfaction by participants and their preference for workshops and discussions, but was unable to evaluate continuing education effectiveness (e.g., relationship to job performance as reported by participating hospital administrators) because of the limitations of the research design.[9]

Although there is a great deal of experience in the field there is a need to collect comparable data about a variety of activities in order to understand the strengths that are available to be built upon in the area of traditional continuing education. This is going to become particularly important in the next year or two. The National Task Force of the National University Extension Association has promulgated the Continuing Education Unit (CEU). The CEU is a unit of measure tentatively defined as "10 contact hours of participation on an organized continuing education, adult or extension experience under responsible sponsorship, capable direction and qualified instruction." The establishment of this unit is an effort to standardize the reporting of such activities in a given institution, between institutions, and in the development and/or assessment of employer and professionally based programs. The CEU will also provide colleges and universities with a basis for reporting their continuing education activities in Full-Time Equivalent (FTE) terms and will create an accounting medium for such activities. The Regional Accrediting Associations will probably adopt it for standardized reporting practices, and possibly for accreditation purposes.

In ideological terms, the development of the CEU represents an acknowledgment that the credit granting system provides access to the degree structure while continuing education structure provides access to certificates. This may be particularly profound for health administration, given the fact that continuing education and health administration are both marginal to the university structure. There is no literature to assist us in dealing with the equation:

health administration $\times$ *continuing education* $=$ *marginality*[2]

Criteria for the development of the CEU are listed below:[10]

> The non-credit activity is planned in response to an assessment of educational need for a specific target population.
>
> There is a statement of objectives and rationale.
>
> Content is selected and is organized in a sequential manner.
>
> There is evidence of pre-planning which should include opportunity for input by a representative of the target group to be served, the faculty area having content expertise, and continuing educational personnel.

The activity is of an instructional nature and is sponsored or approved by an academic or administrative unit of the institution best qualified to affect the quality of the program content and to approve the resource personnel utilized.

There is a provision for registration for individual participants and to provide data for institutional reporting.

Appropriate evaluation procedures are utilized and criteria are established for awarding CEU's to individual students prior to the beginning of the activity. This may include the evaluation of student performance, instructional procedures, and course effectiveness.

Individuals who participate in CEU activities meeting the specified criteria have individual records of their involvement submitted to and will be available from the institution. Continuing Education Units will be assigned to programs in advance and awarded to individual participants who meet the criteria which have been determined in advance for satisfactory completion.

I find it particularly difficult to deal with the substantive differences between these criteria and those which are applied to credit-bearing programs other than the fact that there is a need to create a new higher education currency which is outside of the usual faculty control of the curriculum and the authority to grant credit. There is a need to sort out this new development, given the importance of continuing education to health administration (long-term care particularly). If the CEU becomes a culturally acceptable currency, it may have to link with the career mobility system if not the degree granting system. In either event, the CEU will provide a common currency for in-service or post-entry learning, and has the potential of creating a second hand credentialing system for persons whose ability to achieve career mobility is related to access to continuous learning, which is limited to a credit and/or degree-bearing program. One would hope that there will be a variety of methods for translating the CEU into transferable college credits in order to maximize the openness of the educational system.

Returning to existing continuing education, there does not seem to be any theory of teaching or learning which permeates the educational activity and which acknowledges the adult status of the student body. Most activities seem to be ad hoc and nondevelopmental in the sense that they are not programmed to assist the practitioner to design and complete a sequence of learning activities. (There are several notable exceptions to this.)

For some, continuing education is a continuation of informal job training, for others an updating of formal academic training and for others, the frustrating opportunity to "accumulate enough certificates to paper my office" but not a degree to "handle my status (ego) needs." In neither event "does anyone question my competence because I do a hell of a job." Since status is such an important preoccupation with health administrators, the degree question may have more meaning than the general question of credentialism.

The Concept of Lifelong Learning

Lifelong learning acknowledges the total environment as a learning resource and emphasizes the fact that living is educational experience. It was Confucius, not John Dewey, who wrote:

> "I hear and I forget
> I see and I remember
> I do and I understand"

There are all levels and types of doing, knowing, remembering, and understanding. For an institution, this concept requires acceptance of the fact that personal development and competence can be achieved outside its walls. A responsive institution will demonstrate its willingness to couch its standards, demands and competency requirements in outcome, rather than process terms in order to allow individuals to demonstrate their learning in institutional terms. The acceptance of the concept of lifelong learning has the potential of moving institutions away from preoccupation with process, forces them to clarify their goals and to be accountable for their standards in outcome terms. Behaviorally, a faculty member will no longer have the luxury of returning a major paper with the notation "B–, concepts not fully developed." Faculty will be encouraged and reeducated so that they will be able to state desirable outcomes in terms that have clear meanings to the parties involved and with a pre-agreement about the criteria which will be applied to evaluation.

Acceptance of lifelong learning also can move the educational institution to revise its container-filling theory of distribution requirements. The claim that the undergraduate experience must be four years long in order to get a liberal education is negated by the recognition that the skills of inquiry, and the joy and excitement of learning are the basis for a lifelong pursuit of knowing.

An emerging response to the acceptance of this concept is reflected in the development of undergraduate professional and vocational programs which do not require the traditional liberal education requirements. The concept of lifelong learning (it can be a synonym for continuous education) is being accepted in the context of universal higher education and is buttressed by the needs of colleges and universities to expand their clientele (primarily to adults) and to serve them effectively in an era of increasing accountability and shortage of resources. In specific terms, colleges and universities are responding to the new awareness that more educational activities take place outside their auspices, and that the post-secondary educational era has created a new concept of educational marketing and a new awareness of the "ed biz."

"Almost one-third of America's citizens and almost one-tenth of our GNP are now devoted to education."[11] This conclusion is based on the statistical reports issued by the U.S. Office of Education which indicate the level of participation in elementary, secondary, and higher education. Moses refers to this system as "the Core" (of educational activity).[12] He also develops the concept of "the Periphery"—those educational activities offered in all places where adults are employed, training programs sponsored by voluntary and governmental agencies, instructional television and programs sponsored by proprietary and correspondence schools. "The major criterion for inclusion, 'in the Periphery,' is that these activities involve participation in learning activities through an organized, structured learning situation." The Core and the Periphery make up "The Learning Force" which is defined as "the total number of people developing their capacities through systematic education; that is, where learning is aided by teaching and there are formal, organized efforts to impart knowledge through instruction."[13]

It is estimated that in 1970, 59 million persons were involved in the Core. The data which Moses provides are that approximately 60 million persons were involved in the educational periphery in 1970 and that this figure would leap to 82 million by 1975.[14]

There are no data available which relate the impact of the "periphery" to the GNP.

It is clear, however, that there is a large number of persons receiving educational services which are presumed to increase personal/professional competence, but for which no college credit or degree is awarded. As a result, these persons represent a new "market" for higher education.

Adult Learning and Health Administration Education

There is a variety of theories and approaches to adult learning (Tyler,[15] Knowles,[16] Watson[17]). Each of them acknowledges the importance of identifying the self-concept of adults who see themselves as being capable of self-direction. In addition, they emphasize the role that the adult learner can play in diagnosing learning needs, formulating objectives, planning, designing, implementing learning activities and evaluating results in such a way as to reassess needs, interests, and competency. Self-concept, a well verified sense of self-worth, is important to persons in marginal or "low-status roles." Since the health administrator has a preoccupation with his social status as it affects his job effectiveness, it is particularly important to construct learning environments in which self-concepts are reinforced. In addition, the questions of values are particularly important when we discuss accountability, advocacy, responsiveness, and change agency. "To value is to prefer—There are degrees and levels of preference—What one prefers may be a fact, as opposed to a wish—Conversely what one prefers may be a desired state of affairs and not yet a fact."[18]

If we want to assist the practitioner in evaluating the new behaviors which are being advocated and in creating the desired state of affairs, we need to design an approach in which their negation is equally possible. This suggests the need for a learning environment in which compliance and risk of self and negation are replaced with experimentalism, peer support, and evaluation as feedback. It is difficult, if not impossible, to teach methods of group interaction effectively to a group of 30 through a lecture method. It is equally as impossible to teach independence of judgment in a dependency demanding environment; to teach advocacy in a compliance demanding environment; or to teach accountability in an environment which is not accountable. In each instance, there are role models who are emulated as keys to success. It seems to me that we need to engage in a program of continuous, continuing education for those persons with instructional responsibilities in the field of health administration by providing constant linkage with the problems of contemporary practice on the one hand, and the new knowledge, skills and concepts on the other, to intervene effectively and affect entering and current practitioners. There is a caution, however, as we attempt to convert our preference to a desired state of affairs rather than a wish. As professional persons we turn to our knowledge, expertise, science (or religion) to solve complex problems. When we are disappointed by our inability to dichotomize, simplify or reduce the problem to manageable dimensions, we have a tendency to convert our wants to needs or our desired state of affairs to wishes. We (academics particularly) then construct a set of assumptions (abstractions) with which other persons must live and about which we can contemplate. This survival mechanism of professional people is sometimes labelled as theory building in the academic setting and as a belief in magic or witchcraft in other settings. In either case, it victimizes the persons whom we claim to assist for they must carry the blame for their own humanity. Given our tendency to avoid complex problem solving through a reductionist approach which oversimplifies, or an abstract approach which overgeneralizes, it is small wonder ". . . That a best selling book in America is a fantasy about a seagull who transcends his gullness through the power of positive thinking."[19]

Proposal for the Creation of a National Institute for Health Administration

Based on the preceding analyses, descriptions and discussions, I propose the creation of a National Institute for Health Administration. The purposes of such an Institute are:

1.0 to assure the participation of the existing parties at interest (trade associations, professional associations, AUPHA, etc.);

1.1 to expand the parties at interest to include a variety of consumer interests;

1.2 to create the capability to include new constituencies as the need arises;

1.3 to create a greater sense of accountability *within* the profession;

1.4 (the preceding purposes shall be achieved through the development of a National Advisory Board which shall assist the staff and a Board of Directors in developing priorities and policies);

2.0 to assist the professional associations in developing significant liaison with consumer groups;

2.1 to assist the professional associations in developing a capability for self-assessment, certification and recertification and credentialing of its members;

2.2 to foster interaction between members of the professional groups so as to create a community of interest;

2.3 to assist the professional associations to identify themselves as consumers of educational services;

3.0 (these purposes shall be achieved through the creation of appropriate organizational liaisons, appropriate outside expert capabilities and the Institute staff, and shall include the ability to assess need, and to design, implement, and evaluate);

3.1 to assist the educational service providers to meet the demands of an expanding network of programs and to develop and operate a program of faculty development utilizing Institute members;

3.2 to assist development of an Office of Continuing Education for the field which shall be a repository of information; a source of technical information and assistance; a link to the Institute, its staff capability, membership and team-building capability;

3.3 to develop the capacity to provide college credit and degree granting authority through partnerships, as well as through its own organizational capacity;

3.4 (these purposes shall be achieved by creating a staff capability, and organizational structure which will encourage ad hoc work groups and work teams from its constituency to engage in a variety of developmental activities including program and research applications);

4.0 to provide the staff capability and working relationships with appropriate organizations and individuals to maintain ongoing activities in the definition, development, collection and distribution of the core knowledge and skills necessary to the effective performance of health administration;

4.1 to provide research capability in developing a variety of institutional data, comparative data about full-time and continuing education students, manpower conditions, and patterns of career planning and development;

4.2 to provide a program evaluation capability to the trade and professional associations to develop methods of evaluating program effectiveness;

4.3 to provide a program development capability to the trade and professional associations to develop competency-based approaches to health administrator education;

4.4 to solicit participation in the planning, design, implementation and evaluation of alternative approaches for the education and credentialing of health administrators and to conduct, if necessary, such activities under its own auspices.

ORGANIZATIONAL WORK STRUCTURE

I am proposing a set of porous work groups staffed by an interchangeable set of interdisciplinary persons and led by a team leader who has skills in organization development, team building, as well as his/her substantive area. The interchangeable set of persons will be drawn from the appropriate configuration of participating groups.

Each team will be serviced by a core research group which will be responsible for generating basic data and providing technical assistance to work groups and membership.

Each group will also be serviced by a core training evaluation group which will have the capability of assisting the work group in assessing its progress and in providing technical assistance and training to assist the work group in the achievement of its objectives.

The initial work groups will be Professional Development and Educational Development. These two groups will link with a task group on continuing education and certification.

The work of each of these groups will be coordinated by a council composed of members of each of the active teams, the core groups (evaluation and research) and the task group(s).

Description of Core Groups

1. The Research Group shall be coordinated by a person who is familiar with descriptive and analytic statistics, survey research, computer applications and is familiar with approaches to grounded theory which requires comparative analysis and some model building.

The group shall concentrate its attention on the development of data dealing with characteristics of entering students in health administration programs including attitudinal and value data, socio-economic status and personality data. This program will have to be designed so that participation is voluntary and anonymous and so that the staff will have to defend the request for each cluster of data in terms of its contribution to the field.

Similarly, research will link with other research operations to design a research program to explore patterns of career development of faculty members and practitioners.

Research will also develop a program for getting participation, content, faculty characteristics, et al., data, about continuing education.

2. The Evaluation Group will be coordinated by a person who understands empirical evaluation, assessment of competence and program effectiveness and the provision of analytic descriptions of activity in the context of programmatic goal structures.

Initially the group will explore assessment of some on-going con-

Professional and Educational Development

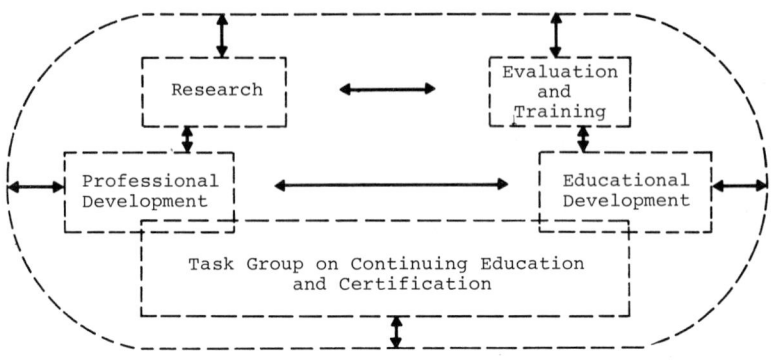

Organizational Governing Structure

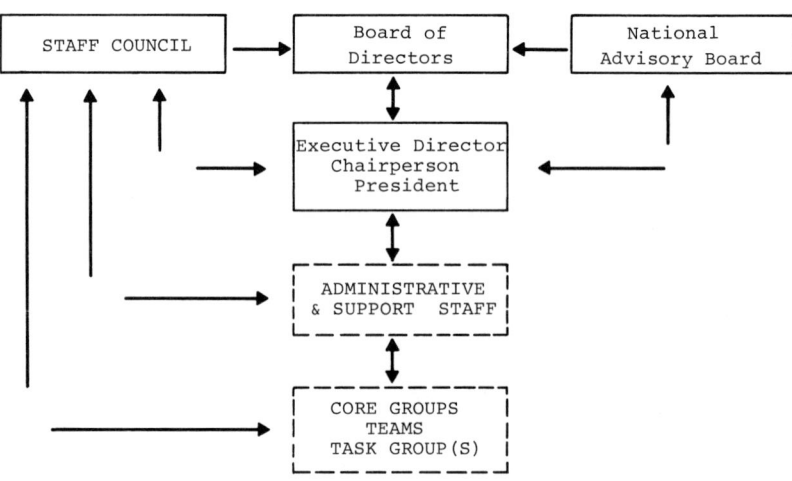

tinuing education activities. The group will also link with the teams to assist in the development of goals, objectives, and a plan of work which can be evaluated.

The evaluation group will combine with the research group and the educational development team with the collaboration of all appropriate groups to design and implement a broad analysis of differentiated role behaviors and skill requirements among health administrators at entry and mid-career levels. The purpose of this inquiry will be to relate the levels of training and education, credentialism and certification to career development and mobility in the field. See Starkweather's 1970 presentation to AUPHA, "A Multi-level Approach to Education for Hospital Administration," for a viewpoint about this matter.

These inquiries will ultimately lead to organizational and curriculum revision at the educational delivery level. (See Appendix A of this paper for Schein's new directions for professional education).[20]

Description of Teams

1. **Professional Development** shall be coordinated by a social scientist with expertise in the development and transition of a profession. The team shall maintain comparative data on activities in other professions and shall assist the team members in developing a liaison with their own organizations. The team will link Team 2 in the Task Group and shall contribute to defining appropriate activities for the role of the professional and trade associations in continuing education and certification. The team shall also link with the Research Group in helping to define needed data about career development. It shall also link with Team 2 in defining appropriate programs for education, credentialing, faculty, and practitioner development.

2. **Educational Development** shall be coordinated by a person with skills in effective program design, implementation and evaluation in a variety of traditional and non-traditional settings. This team will link appropriate participating organizations as well as the Research and Evaluation Core Groups to design:

> A. an Examining College function for the provision of college credit (BA and MA) for experienced practitioners. The team will acknowledge, on one level, the expertise of psychometricians in designing such measures but, on another level, will acknowledge the type of examinations which take place in programs themselves. In light of this awareness, the team will acknowledge the competence of a variety of faculty members and invite pairs/trios of them to develop an examination in their area of competence and to recruit a set of appropriate readers. This program will be instituted quickly and

should provide a needed service to practitioners, and a source of revenue to the Center.

B. a Credit Bank in liaison with the Core Research Groups' computer capability. This credit bank will serve as a repository for credits earned in various ways and will provide transcripts to member colleges and universities who agree to participate in degree-granting or transfer credit arrangements.

C. a Credit Exchange to assist students in translating prior experiences to a common language and credit currency. This function will link to the Examining College function.

D. a Learning Materials Library—there is an array of materials which have been developed at AUPHA member institutions, regional centers, professional and trade associations. These will be gathered, evaluated through liaison with the curriculum evaluation capability of the Evaluation Group. Materials will be made available to interested parties.

E. a variety of alternative educational approaches (correspondence, external degree et al.) to meet the identified and emerging needs of the practicing administrator, entering student and teaching faculty. In this regard intensive linkage will be developed to solicit collaboration in planning and operating new approaches to college credit, degree-granting programs at a B.A., M.A., and Ph.D. level. Team members from professional and trade associations will provide linkage with their associations which might result in co-sponsorship of degree programs by the association(s) and the college(s) and university(ies). Primary emphasis of this endeavor will attempt to meet the needs of the Nursing Home Administrators who are eager to proceed and have the motivation to innovate at the primary level of credentialism and certification.

Conclusion

I recognize the difficulty and possible absurdity of creating such a complex and ambitious national organization. Within this perspective, however, I find it necessary to press for an integrative developmental effort which contains linkage, communication, data, and maximum opportunities for learning.

Obviously, I have come to believe that it is essential to create a new organizational setting in which the accumulated wisdom rooted in the history and traditions of the past can be identified and utilized without being constrained by inherited organizational territoriality, boundary maintenance and the payment of tolls to a variety of gatekeepers. In the process of transformation however, we are sure to create a new set of organizational dilemmas. In this sense, I view the proposal as a value statement constructed as "a desired state of affairs" not yet a fact, but not in realm of wishful thinking or magical belief.

The construction of the Institute is such that it can be developed incrementally with priorities of participants determining the areas to be developed.

This paper has been written as a discussion draft for a group of colleagues to debate, criticize and revise. I have not provided either a budget or a plan for financing the proposed Institute. In this light, I regard this proposal as not complete. I welcome critical reactions to this proposal.

Appendix A

New Directions for Professional Education

The criticisms of the professions and of professional education tend to be the same, whether from the perspective of society, of the professions themselves, or of students entering the professions. They can be summarized as follows:

1. The professions are so specialized that they have become unresponsive to certain classes of social problems that require an interdisciplinary or interprofessional point of view—e.g., the urban problem.
2. Educational programs in professional schools, early career paths, and formal or informal licensing procedures have become so rigid and standardized that many young professionals cannot do the kind of work they wish to do.
3. The norms of entry into the professions have become so rigid that certain classes of applicants such as older people, women, and career switchers are, in effect, discriminated against.
4. The norms of the professions and the growing base of basic and applied knowledge have become so convergent in most professions that it is difficult for innovations to occur in any but the highly specialized content areas at the frontiers of the profession.
5. Professionals have become unresponsive to the needs of many classes of ultimate clients or users of the services, working instead for the organization that employs them.

6. Professional education is almost totally geared to producing autonomous specialists and provides neither training nor experience in how to work as a member of a team, how to collaborate with clients in identifying needs and possible solutions, and how to collaborate with other professionals on complex projects.
7. Professional education provides no training for those graduates who wish to work as members of and become managers of intra- or interprofessional project teams working on complex social problems.
8. Professional education generally underutilizes the applied behavioral sciences, especially in helping professionals to increase their self-insight, their ability to diagnose and manage client relationships and complex social problems, their ability to sort out the ethical and value issues inherent in their professional role, and their ability to continue to learn throughout their careers.

Possible Directions of Reform or Innovation

Direction 1. More flexibility in the professional school curriculum, in the number of paths available through the school, in the number of electives available to students inside and outside the school, in the pacing and sequencing of courses, in the required length of time needed to go through school, and in the degree or certification process used by the school.

Direction 2. More flexibility in the early career paths of professionals, more differentiated rules for licensing to reflect different kinds of professional careers, and more support by the profession itself of role innovation of various kinds.

Direction 3. New curricula and new career paths which are inter- or transdisciplinary and which may lead eventually to new professions that have new blends of knowledge and skill underlying them.

> Meaning 1. A curriculum that involves courses from two or more departments or disciplines leading to a degree named after one of them, or a degree "without specification."
>
> Meaning 2. A curriculum that involves several disciplines, all of which are located within a given school.
>
> Meaning 3. Schools that are from the outset interdisciplinary or transdisciplinary in their orientation in that they set as their goal the development of a new discipline that represents an integration of the disciplines represented.

Direction 4. Complete integration of the behavioral and social sciences into the professional school curriculum at three different levels: (1) basic psychology, sociology, anthropology, and economics as part of the basic science core of professional education; (2) applied behavioral science dealing with the theory and practice of planned change, diagnosis of complex systems, and analysis of client-professional relationships; and (3) applied behavioral science dealing with self-insight, social responsibility, learning how to work in and lead professional teams and learning how to learn.

Notes

1. H. M. Vollmer and D. L. Mills. *Professionalization.* New Jersey: Prentice Hall, 1966.
2. E. H. Schein. *Professional Education.* New York: McGraw-Hill, 1972.
3. Ibid. pp. 8–9.
4. Schein. op. cit. p. 23.
5. Schein. op. cit. p. 24.
6. Schein. op. cit. p. 25.
7. E. C. Hughes. *Men and Their Work.* Glencoe, IL: The Free Press, 1958. p. 129.
8. Schein. op. cit. p. 77.
9. K. J. Matzick. "A National Survey to Evaluate Continuing Education in the Field of Hospital Administration." Health Care Research Series No. 5, University, 1971.
10. Unlabeled CEU mimeographed document, 1973.
11. Roger E. Levien. National Institute of Education: Preliminary Plan for the Proposed Institute, R. 657, HEW. California: Rand Corporation, February 1971.
12. S. Moses. "The Learning Force: A More Comprehensive Program for Education Policy." *Publications in Continuing Education.* Syracuse University. 1971.
13. Ibid.
14. Moses. op. cit.
15. R. W. Tyler. "Academic Excellence and Equal Opportunity." In F. Jarcleroad, ed. *Issues of the Seventies.* San Francisco: Jossey-Bass, 1970.
16. M. Knowles. *The Modern Practice of Adult Education.* New York: Association Press, 1970.
17. G. Watson. "What Do We Know About Learning?" In A. deGrazia and D. Solon, eds. *Revolution in Teaching: New Theory, Technology, and Curricula,* 1964.
18. G. Nettler. "Wanting and Knowing." *American Behavioral Scientist,* October 1973. Vol. 17, No. 1. pp. 5–23.
19. Ibid. p. 22.
20. Schein. op. cit. p. 60 ff.

Health Administration Issues: Implications for Education of Administrators*

Introduction

Health services in the United States—their quantity, quality, distribution, and acceptability—are being questioned today as never before. Significant numbers of providers, of the public, and of the political leadership are adopting the rhetoric of crisis in describing the health system and its problems. The trends operative in the health field have been summarized by Strauss in a paper prepared for the Commission on Education for Health Administration.[1] The author, upon reviewing Strauss' material, reaches a conclusion different from hers. Though the trends she notes are established, and though "disjointed incrementalism" may be the name of the game in this field, trends exist in the social and political environment which will accelerate the rate of change far beyond the modest rate predicted. Indeed, the author believes these environmental changes are sufficient that there will be more fundamental change.

One element of the health crisis is a "crisis of confidence" in the methods for organizing and administering health programs of all types. Here it seems the concern is not mismanagement but nonmanagement. Indeed, the fact that the health system has done as well as it has for as long as it has without the benefits of better-founded administrative efforts is a matter for wonder. Ray Brown took note of this in a recent article when he wrote:

> "An obsession with scientific magic left little place or concern for scientific management. This is not to say that the system did not do well by itself and by the public, as it developed. Actually, it assembled a fabulous set of resources and utilized them in the successful treatment of an exponentially increasing number of patients."[2]

* by James R. Kimmey, M.D., M.P.H.

In his paper, Brown alluded to that which many observers have identified as a prime factor in the failures of health administration in the current health system—the presence of professional domination, particularly by physicians, and the primacy of professional rather than management goals within the system. "Historically," Brown writes, "the system had operated under the spell of medical mystique and under the principle of professional domain." Austin, in his background paper prepared for the Commission stated this problem quite clearly:

> "Since professionals tend to identify more closely with professional goals than with organization, subsystem, or industry goals, the major problems of the health and medical care industry receive minimal attention from the professional groups or their individual members—wherein lies one of the main sources of challenge and opportunity for the emerging health administration profession."[3]

In the author's view, the clearest exposition of the conflict between administrative and professional authority is that of Etzioni.[4] He noted that the role of the administrator in the professional organization, a category including all but proprietary hospitals, is viewed by the professionals as secondary to the organization's major professionally-defined purposes. The administrators deal with the means to support the activities of the organization, while the major goal activities remain completely within professional control. In his discussion, Etzioni identifies three sources of administrators for professional organizations. These sources are: 1) administrators drawn from the ranks of the professions, themselves; 2) graduates of programs in specialized administration which impart understanding of the professional organization to the trainee prior to employment; and 3) lay administrators, who have no training related to the major goal activities of the professional institution or organization. Considering the entire spectrum of organizations subsumed under the definition of "health agency," there are examples of all three types of background represented in chief executive positions. Further, within individual agencies, there are likely to be individuals from all three types of background in positions of significant administrative responsibility. Although these categories were derived to describe an existing situaton, they also have utility in examining options for the future.

In developing an approach to health administration education, attention must be given to the pluralistic nature of the administrative tasks performed in a health setting, and of the backgrounds of individuals performing these tasks. The first part of this paper deals with the author's biases and assumptions concerning health administration. Subsequent sections deal with a structural approach to career education in health administration.

Assumptions and Biases Concerning Health Administration

1. Health administration demonstrates no basic or fundamental differences from other fields of administration. The variations in degree—of complexity, of professionalism, or of values—are not sufficient to justify its classification as unique.

The tendency of knowledge workers in any field of human endeavor to identify the "uniqueness" of their enterprise is well established. The establishment of the unique characteristics of a field which set it apart from all related or unrelated societal activities is an important first step on the road to professional status for its practitioners.

The uniqueness of health administration as a field is implied in the majority of articles on the subject appearing in *Hospital Administration,* the journal of the American College of Hospital Administrators, and in the various publications of the Association of University Programs in Health Administration. As long as the uniqueness remains implicit, it is difficult to challenge. Two efforts to make explicit the uniqueness of the field are found in recent literature. The first, in a report on graduate education for health administration in the United States by Professor Teddy Chester[5] defines several characteristics differentiating hospital administration from other administrative endeavors. The second, in Austin's paper prepared for the Commission,[6] offers a set of characteristics defining uniqueness of health administration generally.

The characteristics identified by Chester as differentiating hospital administration from other areas of administration were challenged by Westfall in the MacEachern Memorial Lecture of the American College of Hospital Administrators in 1969.

> The first characteristic identified was that hospital service and customers are different. Services are highly technical and are consumed away from home. The consumer does not have the choice of when he consumes hospital services; he consumes when he is sick and is required to go to a hospital. A mechanic might point out that one could describe a man who is having trouble with his auto in the same terms. He needs a technical service; he hasn't chosen the time at which he needs it—it has been forced upon him; and he is going to consume it at some place away from home. In other

words, this "unique characteristic" of hospital service is not really a basic difference but a superficial one.

A second characteristic that was presumed to distinguish hospitals from other institutions was that the producers of hospital services—the doctors—are highly skilled professionals who are difficult to handle. Those who have been in academic administration for any period of time will say the same description applies to philosophy. The typical businessman who has a research and development department staffed with Ph.D.'s in chemistry and physics undoubtedly has the same problem, and James Webb, or his successor at NASA, has the same difficulty with the Wernher von Brauns and the like. This is no fundamental difference.

Another difference suggested by this study was that administrators of hospitals have a large and diffuse educational job. They train people at low levels of skill and people in highly technical jobs. How much difference arises in this respect between the hospital administrator's job and that of the business excutive who has the responsibility of training men to take over the chief executive's spot and at the same time must train people who have such a low degree of skill that they haven't even been in the job market up to now?

A fourth characteristic that was said to distinguish the hospital administrator was the manner in which he was held accountable. The hospital administrator is accountable to a board, but there are no clear-cut standards for judging good hospital administration. It is difficult to say that this hospital administrator is doing a good job, and that one, a bad job. Undoubtedly, that is true. Educators, however, are equally at sea when it comes to evaluating their results. In fact, it is difficult to define exactly what the educator is supposed to do. What would be the description of a proper product when the educators are through? Again, I think a distinction of this sort is more superficial than fundamental.

The final distinction that was made in this particular study was that the hospital administrator has an unusual public relations job. He has to raise money from the same people whom he charges for the services that he provides. Again, it would be hard to find a university president who doesn't feel he has exactly the same problem.[7]

Westfall's arguments against uniqueness seem to have merit. The same generic types of administrative problems are present in other situations. Some may be relatively more important in the health organization setting than in the shoe factory, but some things that are very important in administering the shoe factory are of relatively little importance in the hospital. The point is that there are degrees of difference between hospital administration and other kinds of administration, but not a set of unique characteristics setting hospital administration apart.

The same comment seems valid in reviewing Austin's description of the features of the health and medical care industry which contribute to the uniqueness of health administration (which would include hospital administration). It seems presumptuous to claim that the delivery of individualized services, or the problems of professionalism, or the problem of complexity within the industry are unique to health. Indeed, Austin anticipates that some would disagree. To the extent that these factors differ in a health organization—as viewed from the perspective of administration—they are quantitative and not qualitative descriptors.

One factor which neither Chester nor Austin attempted to use as a descriptor of the uniqueness of health administration is the value system reflected in our traditional approach to public and institutional health services. This formulation, to which I might have subscribed four or five years ago, would hold that the life and death nature of the end product of the health industry as well as the service orientation of both the personnel and institutions constituted a qualitative difference between health and other fields and therefore a unique characteristic. Suspicion grows that even this difference is one of degree, and as physicians organize in trade unions, nurses and other health workers strike for higher wages, and hospitals threaten to close, if forced to comply with community planning, the degree of difference lessens. The foregoing contributes to the conclusion, then, that the similarity of skills, knowledge, and techniques required for management of health enterprises as compared to nonhealth enterprises are infinitely greater than the differences among such enterprises.

2. There is insufficient data to support any hypothesis concerning the efficacy of one or another track—e.g., combination of formal education, training, and/or experience—in preparing "successful" health administrators.

One of the major stumbling blocks in the way of studying health administration is the lack of complete and/or relevant historical or current data. The majority of the studies in the literature are either out-of-date, or restricted in their scope to one class of administrative manpower, the hospital executive. This places the observer—be he perpetuator, revisionist, iconoclast, or scientist—in a different position. Who are the health administrators? How did they prepare for their work? Where are they employed? How much do they earn? What are the characteristics of success? The seminal research question "What is health administration?" is answered satisfactorily in Austin's definition:

302

Health administration is planning, organizing, directing, controlling, coordinating, and evaluating the resources and procedures by which needs and demands for health and medical care and a healthful environment are fulfilled, by the provision of specific services to individual clients, organizations, and communities.[8]

In the context of such a global definition, however, the problem of adequate data is intensified. Not only do we lack concrete information on the types of organizations in which health administration is practiced, but the majority of studies available concentrate on the top line administrator and take little note of the others involved in administrative decision making in a specific health setting.

Within the past year, three authors have proposed a broad classification for health administrative personnel. The three schemes presented are interesting for their similarities as well as for the conclusions drawn by the authors. Austin suggests four broad categories: health care statesman, organizational executive, middle management personnel, and administrative staff specialist.[9] Brown suggested the following typology (reordered for consistency with Austin's classification): policy makers; executives; functionaries; researchers, and planners.[10] Finally, Stallones suggested categorization under three classes: health and medical care statesmen; agency directors and their surrogates, present and projected; and personnel administrators, business managers, and the like.[11] All three authors differentiated among these categories in terms of desirable background and preparation. Although hierarchy was implied by each, vertical mobility was not. Austin and Stallones concluded that the area of concentration for the Commission on Education for Health Administration should fall in the category of organizational executive/agency director. This conclusion will be discussed below.

Even with the simple categorization of administrative personnel proposed by these three authors, information necessary to analyze relative roles, mobility, and appropriate training is not currently available.

The whole matter of the data base for studying health administration manpower was examined in a comprehensive fashion by Ruchlin and his colleagues.[12] This paper summarized and commented upon the body of existing literature in hospital administration manpower research. It makes worthwhile reading. Of particular importance to the Commission on Education for Health Administration is their epilogue in which the author would concur:

The proliferation of graduate programs and the emergence of undergraduate programs in health care administration coupled with similar developments in the public health field have elicited fears that the evolution of educational programs has proceeded based on internally generated rather than externally catalyzed momentum. While the realization is widespread that new directions are mandatory in the realm of educational planning, and while a few preliminary steps have been taken in this direction, the fact remains that the knowledge base required for such educational planning is scant.[13]

My bias would suggest that the most valid intermediate-range recommendation of the Commission would be that adequate resources be invested in research in the field before additional resources are invested in existing programs or in new models that may represent more internally generated change for the sake of change.

3. A far greater number of internal management decisions affecting the output and effectiveness of any health organization are made by individuals with no formal training in health administration than by trained health administrators, a situation unlikely to change appreciably in the immediate future.

One of the characteristics of management in the health setting which may distinguish it from other settings is the degree to which individuals with health professional training rather than administrative training occupy line positions. In the typical corporation, staff departments are often headed by professionals exercising administrative responsibilities within their departments, such as the scientist-administrator in research and development. Line positions, on the other hand, are typically occupied by individuals with management training but without a particular specialty or another professional identification. In the health organization, it is much more likely that key line management positions such as director of nursing, chief pharmacist, director of environmental health, or coordinator of community outreach services, are occupied by individuals with professional preparation in their field but relatively little formal management training. These individuals may have substantial ability as administrators which they have developed through experience and, given the opportunity and technical tools, could generalize to a broader segment of the health organization. Yet these individuals are not a substantial pool of sorely-needed general administrative talent unless they are willing to return to school at mid-career and "get their union card" in the form of an MPH, and MHA, or other credential attesting to their ability as managers. If they are unable, for a variety of reasons, to undertake such additional training, they are then topped-out on their career ladder and subjected to the frustrations of the salary differentials between their categorical management job and the generalized management job of the assistant administrator of the institution or agency.

Proceeding from this prejudice, one is distressed when Austin, speaking for the Commission states: "We have chosen to focus on (organizational executives) and to place primary emphasis on the study of educational strategies designed to prepare entrants into the field of health administration who aspire to the role of organizational executive at some point in their careers."[14] It is not difficult to read into this—supported by some knowledge of the behavior of professions—a growing effort to reserve the role of organizational executive to individuals who have undergone one type of training, who have obtained prerequisites of professional status in health administration, and who have "gone through the chairs" as determined by the gatekeepers of the profession.

An adverse reading of Brown leads to an even more unacceptable conclusion. He defines executives as "those whose primary responsibility is for the performance of others . . . the line officers."[15] He then goes on to define sufficient training programs for executives in health settings as follows:

> The program sufficient for the training of hospital executives can serve appropriately for the training of all health services management executives requiring general management training. If such a program effectively meets the requirements for the training of the hospital executive, its products can effectively meet the training requirements for all executives in the health field. The hospital represents the most complex management situation in the health field, and it also has the most complex set of external relationships of any agency or enterprise in the field.[16]

This might suggest the reverse of the blocked career ladder, e.g., that all line administrative positions should be filled by graduates of hospital administration programs, thus completing the parallel (and often competitive) administrative and professional structures that already plague the top levels of health organizations.

This leads to another point.

4. The further professionalization of health administration has no proven utility and may be counter productive.

One of the consistent themes running through the discussion of health administration cited elsewhere in this paper has been the negative effect of health professionalism on administration in health organizations. Yet implicit in suggestions for future training for health administration is the idea that by professionalizing health administration the adverse effects of professionalism can be overcome. In the author's view, it is naive to assume that the health administration profession will be motivated to behave in any way different from the twenty-five or so existing and identified health professions, and that it alone will be guided by "responsiveness, responsibility, and reconciliation."[17] In this context, it also seems presumptuous for the professionists to suggest that administrators may be the logical chosen group within the health system which can pull it together.[18] In the author's view, better administration in the health field can make a difference—it can pull together. It makes little difference, however, whether this improved management is carried out by administrative professionals or professional administrators. In the real world of the seventies, it will have to be both.

An Approach to Health Administration Career Education

A number of articles trace the development of health administration and health administration training in the United States.[19] All of the training efforts, though varying widely in auspices, academic requirements, practice requirements, and degrees granted, seem to this observer to have attempted to do two things. First, they have attempted to equip the student with the technical tools and concepts of administration. Second, they have attempted to inculcate a set of values appropriate to the student's career choice of health administration. Recognizing that it is a generalization and may not reflect the specifics of 1970s situation, it seems that over time two different approaches to health administration training have tended to grow up in two different environments. Programs oriented to training of public health administrators have developed within schools of public health and have more often than not attracted students with professional preparation in a health discipline. Such programs seek to equip these health professionals with the values and techniques of management and administration before sending them back to the world of practice. Programs designed to prepare hospital administrators have tended to grow up in a variety of academic settings (schools of public health, schools of business, schools of health administration, etc.). These programs accept greater numbers of individuals without professional preparation in health and are designed to impart to them the values and techniques of management and administration as well as the values of health.

Thus functioning models exist both for the preparation of administrative professionals and of professional administrators for the health field.

It seems clear from a reading of the variety of editorials and articles in this general field (some of which are cited above) that there are pressures for consolidating administrative training into a single model and professionalizing health administration. This has lead to a polarization to some extent between the Association of University Programs in Health Administration representing the second type of program and the Association of Schools of Public Health representing, broadly, the first. Jurisdictional disputes and adoption of win-lose attitudes by either or both of the groups can only delay development of a solution to the pressing problem of improving health administration as it is practiced in the United States. The deliberations and conclusions of the Commission on Education for Health Administration, and the degree to which follow up activities are developed, cannot help but affect the outcome of this dispute. For purposes of a theoretical discussion, one might establish a continuum between two polar positions. At one end would be the position that all health administrators should be drawn from the ranks of health professionals because only health professionals understand the special problems and the value structure of the health system. At the other extreme, the position would be that administration of health services should be placed completely in the hands of professional managers because the health system is really no different from any other socio-economic system and will respond to the practice of good management principles. Conventionally, having established such a continuum, one would say the answer lies somewhere in the middle. It does not. It does not because the continuum (and its polar statements) is not relevant to the problem. Given the definition of health administration cited earlier in this paper, the problem—for society, for the practitioner, for the educator, and for the Commission— is to improve the quality of administrative decision-making and practice at *every* level in *every* component of the health system. The concern is essentially pragmatic: does the system work? In the author's view, securing a positive answer is more dependent on the quality of administrative practice throughout the system than at any selected level.

For purposes of developing a new approach to education for health administration, the following goal statement has been formulated:

> The goal of health administration career education is to improve the efficiency and effectiveness of the health system in delivering its services to

people through improved management at every level of the resources available for carrying out the system's tasks.

This goal statement has a number of implications for any approach to education for health administration designed to meet its requirements. First, the approach should concern itself with health administration *career* education in the sense of being a continuous process throughout the individual administrator's career. It cannot, and should not, be measured by a single educational experience at the entry point into an administrative career. Second, the concern of a new approach to education for health administration should encompass all health workers with management responsibilities rather than those who aspire to a single role, top administrator. In terms of systemic effectiveness, the best trained and most competent chief executive officer cannot compensate for inadequate managerial skills at other levels in the organization which he heads. Third, a new approach to education for health administration should emphasize opportunities for career mobility, both horizontal and vertical, to administrators who are concentrating on health, or to health professionals concentrating on administration. Fourth, the approach should provide a mechanism for stimulating and motivating individuals in administrative positions to improve their knowledge of the tools and techniques of administration continuously. Finally, because of the current problems with quantity and quality in administration, the approach should provide a mechanism for assisting those already in the field as well as those coming to the field in the future.

Elements of the Model

This proposal for improving the overall quality of health administration practice is oriented to structure rather than content of education and training programs for health administrators. In the author's view, health administrators will continue to come into the field from a variety of backgrounds, and such diversity is desirable. It also seems desirable that heterogeneity of formal education programs, particularly those offering advanced degrees, be promoted. The approach presented here would avoid the imposition of the minimum requirement or core curriculum as the measure of acceptability of an educational program, and attempts to give weight to the major factor in the art as opposed to the science of management, i.e., experience. It is, without apology, an attempt to stem the tide of professionalization of health administration, substituting instead a broad recognition, through the registration process, of the large numbers of individuals in the field who exercise administrative responsibilties. It is hoped that this approach might stimulate this larger group to improve its understanding of the basic principles and tools of administration, and to keep abreast of changes in the field. In the author's view, the most important aspect of the proposed approach is its establishment of an organized framework for career development of administrative talent for the health field, both within institutions and throughout the system. In another context, it has been suggested that the educational institutions assume this responsibility for career coordination that might be considered as an alternative to the present proposal.[20] It seems imperative that some mechanism for such coordination be developed if the goal stated earlier is to be achieved.

NATIONAL HEALTH ADMINISTRATION CAREER DEVELOPMENT PROGRAM

I recommend that a new national program be established under the auspices of a non-profit corporation to coordinate the basic and continuing education of health administrators, and to provide recognition of individuals who attain, and maintain, a specified level of educational preparation while functioning as administrators in a health setting. (See Appendix I) The program has three elements:

1. The Organizational Career Development Program (OCDP) providing basic management training on an in-service basis to the administrative employees of health organizations and institutions in a defined area.

2. The Academic Career Development Program (ACDP) providing advanced courses and degree work in administration and management to full- and part-time students.

3. The National Health Administration Career Development Registry providing a mechanism for recognizing achievement of educational and experience goals in health administration, and for motivating administrators to maintain their proficiency.

A number of formal and informal relationships among these elements could evolve. The one consistent factor binding the elements would be the granting of career development credits to participating administrative personnel based on their participation in educational activities conducted under OCDP or ACDP auspices.

Organizational Career Development Program

Under this proposal, health organizations employing administrators —which is to say all health organizations—would join to establish a formal organizational career development program for those administrators. The method for determining the level at which OCDP's would be established might vary with the size and number of health organizations in an area. Depending on the population, numbers of institutions, and numbers of personnel, OCDP's might be organized on a community, areawide or state basis. It would be important that different types of health organizations participate in the same OCDP and its educational offerings. Organizational models such as comprehensive health planning areas and regional medical program subregions are suggested as possibilities. Each OCDP should establish a formal relationship with an academic program in management in an institution or institutions in its servce area (not necessarily an ACDP).

The OCDP would organize and conduct basic courses in the fields of financial management, personnel management, information processing, administrative practice, and planning. Faculty for the program would be drawn from participating, operating, and academic institutions, and academic credit might or might not be given depending on arrangements with the affiliated academic institution. Career development credits would be given for satisfactory completion of these courses, based on the relative value scale discussed below.

Participation in the courses would be open to all employees of participating health organizations and institutions, subject to approval of their supervisor. Institutions will be expected to stress each supervisor's responsibility for developing his or her line subordinate's knowledge and ability in administration. The OCDP would report annually to the registry (see below on the career development credits earned by individuals in participating institutions.

Academic Centers for Health Administration Career Education

In the context of this approach to health administration career education, the academic center is conceived as an interdepartmental program within a major university offering the following types of educational experience in the broad field of health administration:

1. Doctoral programs for individuals with career objectives of research or broad policy-making roles in health administration.

2. Master's degree programs in management with a health orientation. As is presently the case, candidates for these degrees may or may not have previous health professional training. In order to provide maximum flexibility for candidates for the master's degree they should be offered in two settings.

First, a full-time academic program for students in residence, and *Second,* an external degree program to permit individuals employed full-time in health administration (or other areas) to complete the master's degree requirements through course work taken at institutions other than the academic center approved by the center for that purpose.

3. Develop and coordinate the offering of non-degree continuing education courses in health administration which may be offered by the individual centers or by consortia of centers on a national, regional, state, or district basis.

4. Work with OCDP's in development of curricula and course materials for their localized basic training efforts.

The National Health Administration Career Development Registry

A key feature in this approach to health administration career education is the establishment of a health administration career development registry at the national level. This registry would be a nonprofit corporation guided by corporate members and directors representing professional organizations, provider organizations, OCDP's, academic centers, and consumer interests. The registry would exist for the sole purpose of maintaining a current record of the career development credits earned by each registrant involved in health administration from in-service training, academic training, and/or experience. The registry would perform the following functions:

1. Identify the various positions within health organizations of all types exercising administrative responsibility.

2. Establish a relative value scale for various types of educational activities and health administration experiences.

3. Maintain a listing (registry) of health workers in an administrative career track who: a) offer a specified minimum number of career development credits at the time of initial application for registration, and b) offer a specified number of additional career development

credits at specified time intervals as a condition of continued registration.

4. Monitor the entire system for health administration career development and periodically report on its status.

Career Development Credits and the Relative Value Scale

A major goal of the proposed approach to education for health administration is to shift the emphasis from "gatekeeper" credentialling to development and maintenance of knowledge of management principles and practice. In the author's opinion, this requires that recognition be given to a variety of types of educational and operational experience which contribute to the development of an effective administrator. If a registry approach is to be used to achieve this, then a methodology must be developed for weighting both educational activities of varying complexity and experiences in different types of administrative settings. It is proposed that initial registration as a registered health administrator (RHA) require a certain number of career development credits and continued registration also be dependent on credits earned on the basis of current experiences and training activities. One of the major tasks facing the registry would be the establishment of a relative value scale. (Appendix II to this paper suggests how the scale would work. The establishment and acceptance of the relative value scale would be an essential initial function of the registry board at the time of implementation of the program.)

Summary

An approach to education for health administration has been suggested which has the following characteristics: 1) it retains a great deal of flexibility for academic programs designed to prepare individuals to assume responsible management positions in the health services industry; 2) it institutionalizes in-service training and continuing education for individuals functioning as administrators in a health setting; 3) it provides a number of options for individuals functioning as administrators who are motivated to maintain a high degree of understanding of the current trends in their field; 4) it provides opportunities for formal training in administration to individuals in operating institutions and agencies who might not otherwise have such an opportunity without leaving the work force for a prolonged period; 5) it provides recognition of the importance of both education and experience in developing and maintaining administrative capacity.

In the author's opinion, this program lends itself to demonstration on a limited basis, a state or region, while its effectiveness is evaluated. Such a demonstration could proceed concurrently with essential data gathering on health administration personnel which is felt to be required for meaningful long range policy recommendations and decisions.

Appendix I
NATIONAL HEALTH ADMINISTRATION CAREER DEVELOPMENT PROGRAM

Form of Organization

A new national organization would be established as a non-profit corporation under the laws of a convenient state. The corporate structure would be conventional, with a corporate membership electing a board to carry out the corporate businesses. The board would establish such committees and hire such staff as required to carry out the program. The organization of the membership and constitution of the board would be designed to secure participation of the groups involved in health administration career development.

Corporate Members

The following groups are suggested as classes of organization that should participate in the governance of the program:

- National professional organizations of health administrators, or which have significant numbers of health administrators among their membership
- National associations of health institutions and agencies employing health administrators
- National associations of educational institutions or programs engaged in training health administrators

Board of Directors

Members of the board would be elected to represent specific elements in the total program. A possible distribution might be:

- Three representatives of organizations of administrators
- Three representatives of institutions and agencies employing administrators

- Three representatives of Academic Centers
- Three representatives of Organizational Career Development Programs
- Four representatives-at-large not otherwise identified with the previously enumerated groups

Appendix II

RELATIVE VALUE SCALE AND CAREER DEVELOPMENT CREDITS

A. Excerpts from a Relative Value Scale †

Category	Type of Education or Experience	Unit	Relative Value/Unit
Acad.	Grad. level course work in mgt. or related field at an Academic Center or certified by such a Center	Cr.	1.00
"	Grad. level course work in mgt. or related field offered in a continuing education program by an Academic Center or certified by a Center	Cr.	1.00
"	Undergrad. level course work in mgt. or related field	Cr.	0.75
In-serv.	OCDP course with academic credit	Cr.	0.50
"	OCDP course without academic credit	Hr.	0.01
Experience	Administrative Level I ††	Yr.	10.00
"	" " II	Yr.	9.00
"	" " III	Yr.	8.50
"	" " V	Yr.	6.00
"	" " IX	Yr.	1.50

† Numerical values assigned are for demonstration purposes only.

†† Administrative levels would be defined by the board on the basis of review of complexity of various administrative positions in health agencies, with Level I representing the highest level of complexity.

B. Application to a Case

The board would have to decide what level of career development credits would be required for initial registration and what level would be required during a finite period for re-registration. For purposes of the example, assume the following:

- 30 career development credits for initial registration
- 10 career development credits each 3 years for re-registration, which must include at least two types of credits from the relative value scale categories

Smith, John P.

Item		No. of Units	Rel. Value/Unit	C. D. Credits
B.S. (Biology)	1961	0		
M.A. (Hosp. Adm.)	1964	30	1.00	30
M.P.H. (Adm.)	1970	30	1.00	30
Dr.P.H. (Adm.)	1972	30	1.00	30
			Subtotal Acad.	90
Hospital office mgr. 61–62		1	1.50	1.50
Adm. Asst. 290 bed hosp. 64–65		1	3.00	3.00
Asst. Adm., 290 bed hosp. 65–66		1	5.00	5.00
Asst. Adm., 415 bed hosp. 66–69		3	7.00	21.00
V–P 600 bed hosp. 72–73		1	9.00	9.00
			Subtotal Exp.	39.50
			Total	129.50

If the registry had been active, Smith would have been registered in 1964 on the basis of 31.5 cumulative C.D. points. He would have been re-registered in 1967 on the basis of 15 additional points, and in 1970 with 44 additional credits, and in 1973 with 39 additional points. At this level, he will accumulate at least 27 experience points by 1976, but would have to present at least 1 education credit as well to retain registration.

Notes

1. Janet A. Strauss. "Future Trends in Health Care Delivery, A Forecast." Washington, D.C.: Commission on Education for Health Administration, August 1973.
2. Ray Brown. "Training for Health Service Management." *Hospital Administration*, Summer 1973. Vol. 18, No. 3. p. 13.
3. Charles J. Austin. "What is Health Administration?" Washington, D.C.: Commission on Education for Health Administration, October 1973. p. 4.
4. Amitai Etzioni. *Modern Organizations*. Englewood Cliffs, NJ: Prentice Hall, 1964. pp. 75 ff.

5. Theodore E. Chester. *Graduate Education for Hospital Administration in the United States.* Chicago: American College of Hospital Administrators, 1969.
6. Austin. op. cit. p. 23.
7. Ralph Westfall. "Educating for the Future." *Hospital Administration,* Summer 1969. Vol. 14, No. 3. pp. 81 ff.
8. Austin. op. cit. p. 23.
9. Austin. op. cit. pp. 15–16.
10. Brown. op. cit. pp. 16–17.
11. Reuel A. Stallones. Unpublished notes prepared for the Commission on Education for Health Administration, October 1973. p. 2.
12. Hirsch R. Ruchlin, Dennis D. Pointer, and Samuel Levey. "Health Administration Manpower Research: A Critique and a Proposal." *Hospital Administration,* Summer 1973. Vol. 18, No. 3. pp. 81 ff.
13. Ibid. p. 104.
14. Austin. op. cit. p. 16.
15. Brown. op. cit. p. 16.
16. Brown. op. cit. p. 19.
17. Strauss. op. cit. pp. 46–47.
18. Austin. op. cit. p. 24.
19. See for example:
    Jon B. Jaeger. *Education for Health Administration: A Conceptualization.* Chicago: Center for Health Administration Studies. 1973. p. 1–2; and Solomon J. Axelrod. "A Historical View of the Teaching of Medical Care Administration." *American Journal of Public Health.* Supplement I, Volume 59, January 1969. pp. 61–66.
20. James R. Kimmey. "Letter to the Editor." *American Journal of Public Health,* May 1971. Vol. 61, No. 5. pp. 895–897.

The Organizational Network of Education for Health Administration*

Introduction

The Commission's intent for this paper is different from others of the eight. Each of the others deals with some substantive issue in health administration education and practice, while this one deals with the organizational mechanism by which issues may be approached. To an important degree, structure dictates how various activities will be performed; enhancing some, obscuring some, and modifying still others. Thus, organization has a fundamental effect on most questions which the Commission has addressed. Further, it is important to any implementation of the Commission's ideas.

As requested, the approach taken herein will be normative. Further, it will attempt to be broad, dealing not only with the *inter*-structure among educational programs, but also the *extra*-structure of this network relative to its environments.

The framework for this paper is contained in Figure 1. The three dimensions of the figure will be discussed first, followed by particular comment on several clusters of cells which are derived from the three. Specific proposals will be interspersed throughout.

Degree of Concentration, Present and Proposed

The pattern of horizontal relationships among faculty groups can be placed on a spectrum which runs from complete *dispersion*—no formal relationships—to complete *integration*—virtually all collaborative efforts are channeled and controlled from a single organizational

* by David B. Starkweather

FIGURE 1

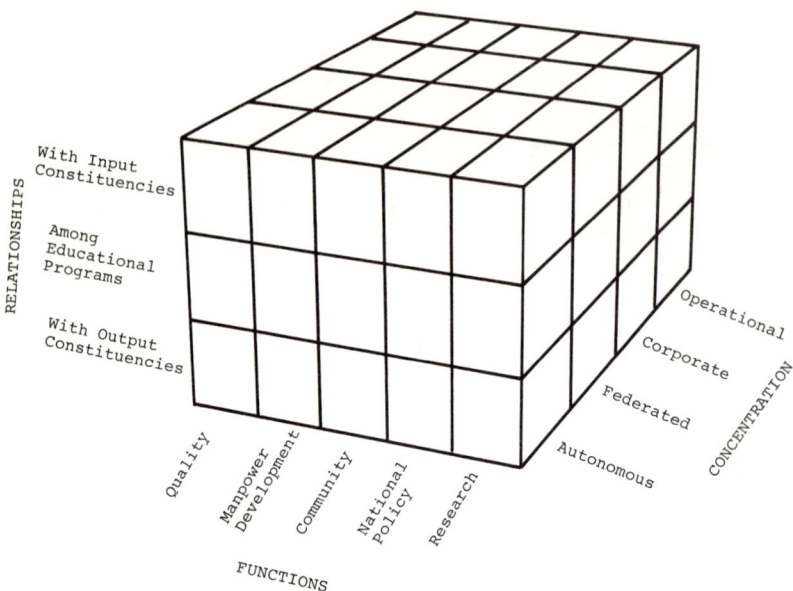

source. Between these hypothetical extremes there is a rather broad range of possible patterns. Real organizations of educational venture such as health administration seem to fall into four categories:

Autonomy: faculties and programs give only limited credence to associational effort, nurturing and guarding instead the prerogatives of independent academic effort. The prime advantages would appear to be maximization of educational innovation and variety, and minimal financial burden. Associations in this category are "reluctant dean's clubs." Examples in health and medical education are the Association of Schools of Public Health (until very recently) and the Association of Teachers of Preventive Medicine.

Federation: facilities and programs voluntarily give over certain functions to a commonly held association, expecting the association to represent their interests and to undertake shared activities. An example is the American Association of Medical Colleges prior to its reorganization in the late sixties following the Coggeshall Report.

Incorporation: going beyond representation and sharing of commonly held viewpoints and activities, the organization actively modifies and molds the long run and even short run character of effort by urging and forcing new efforts and abandoning old ones. The organization assumes a life of its own, and tension develops within it between activities which "serve the members" and those which "lead the way." The post-Coggeshall AAMC is an example of this type.

Operational: the association assumes operation responsibility for delivery of education, in effect taking over activities usually located on campuses. There is no complete example of this currently at hand, but portions of it exist with organizations such as the Educational Testing Service, centralized admitting plans, certain educational consortia, the National Intern Matching Plan and National Boards of AAMC, and credentialling and continuing education efforts of national professional societies.

The principal organization in health administration education is the Association of University Programs in Health Administration. It stands between "federation" and "incorporation" on this spectrum, with strong momentum in recent years from the former to the latter. Some of its characteristics are:

- Well established and well funded from multiple sources
- Broad participation of member institution faculty, going well beyond program directors
- Active development of curriculum materials and other services to members
- Precise membership and participation provisos, and relatively small policy-setting body
- Strong secretariat
- Action and activity oriented: capable of mounting numerous and varied tasks and bringing them to conclusion
- Tradition of hospital orientation, which is incomplete view of the total scope of health administration.

A second view of the dispersion-concentration spectrum is one of vertical relationships between the health administration educational establishment and professional and institutional groups in the practicing world; "town-gown" rather than "gown-gown" relationships. This is influenced, in turn, by the "town-town" organization within the professional community. Concerning this latter, there is dispersion in some sectors and relative concentration in others. In the realm of health facilities and services administration, the dispersion runs to several institutional membership associations—notably American Hospital Association, and American Federation of Hospitals and American Nursing Home Association—and several separate personal membership societies—American College of Hospital Administrators, American College of Nursing Home Administrators, Association of Mental Health Administrators, etc. By contrast, in the realm of public health the institutional and personal membership organization is one: American Public Health Association. In the work of business administration there is marked separation and proliferation of both institutional and personal membership groups.

As for the town-gown structure, there is relatively more integration of effort and power in public health (for instance, APHA still operates the accreditation program for schools of public health, and there is substantial involvement of school of public health deans and faculty in APHA), relatively less in health facilities and services administration (the school accreditation function is separate from both AHA and ACHA, and there is now minimal involvement of program directors and faculty in these organizations), and in the business world there are no formal town-gown links.

These relationships can be restated as follows:

Public health: With the professional community highly integrated, it seemed in the past unnecessary for the academic community to organize itself. But now this is seen as increasingly important. With this gown-gown structuring will come a greater town-gown distinction.

Health facilities and services administration: With the professional community somewhat dispersed, the academic community has become organized, probably in an attempt to span in academic outlook what is not bridged in practice. There have developed town-gown distinctions.

Business administration: Both practicing and academic community are dispersed.

These three sets of structures are the ones which impinge most directly on the scope of the Commission's responsibility, and they lead to the following issues.

Should the health administration education field become rationalized? Academics in the field are fond of designing models for rationalized health care delivery, to which practicing administrators sometimes respond: "get your own house in order." The recent development of undergraduate programs, coupled with the continuing mess in continuing education, has inspired much discussion but little real accomplishment at vertical integration (as compared to horizontal links among graduate programs operating at the master's degree level).

Conceptually, a strong argument can be made that such should not take place: that diversity and innovation are stifled by organization of the educational establishment. Support for this argument is summarized in the minutes of a recent Commission meeting:

> He (C. Austin) characterized existing programs as follows: a) there are probably enough programs *in toto,* but they are quite uniform in character and too few focus on new markets, using non-traditional approaches, or developing research capabilities; b) there is possibly a need for a large center of excellence; c) programs are now in a variety of university settings and this is OK provided there is access to all university resources; and d) the programs' credibility is low for several reasons—small size, faculty weaknesses, and poor research capability.[1]

It's not at all clear that these weaknesses can be laid to the organizational network which has developed among the programs, primarily AUPHA and Accreditation Commission for Graduate Education in Hospital Administration. These organizations have not directly stimulated the recent proliferation of new programs. The increasing variety of university settings, and notably the multi-departmental sponsorship of several new programs (e.g., University of Washington group degree), is probably the result in part of both AUPHA consultation as well as ACGEHA standards. Questions of insufficient size and research capacity may have resulted from accreditation standards that indicated that low minimums in these areas were sufficient. The question of uniformity is most troublesome. Slavish conformity, obtained in part through a network of communication which allows faculty at one setting to "do what Charlie is doing" simply because it is easy to ascertain and fits a subtle but powerful set of informal norms, is truly antithetical to what universities are all about.

On the other hand, several of the academic ills proposed above can be laid directly to universities: rushing into an educational field without adequate preparation and without the necessary faculty skills; reaching for soft money funding rather than using basic university sources; and responding too readily to here-and-now job markets rather than to the longer run systemic needs of the health field.

On balance, it appears that the impact of these problems on existing programs in health administration education has been noticeable and significant—sometimes direct but often subtle—and that whatever errors have been made are more of omission than commission: failure to establish higher threshold standards for new programs (granting that to do so would have invited charges of AMA-type structuring; and some lack of stimulus to innovation as compared to conformity to group norms.

A strong argument can also be made that the organizational network should be strengthened and expanded. The argument rests on several points: (1) the continuing need for public funding, which demands constant, aggressive and well-coordinated Washington representation; (2) the need to establish higher standards of educational quality coupled with assistance to universities in attaining such quality by stimulating the development of qualified faculty, advising on academic structure, developing effective curricula, and stimulating research; (3) the need to undertake certain collective functions such as recruitment of new kinds and qualities of students; and (4) the need to develop and modify national policies which bear on health administration education.

In short, there needs to be a well developed organization of the broadest possible scope, but there also needs to be a way in which such organization avoids stultifying influence. **The Commission should: (1) support selective strengthening and expansion of the organizations in the field of health administration education, (notably AUPHA, but not limited to it); and (2) seek implementation of mechanisms whereby such further development will contain self-correction, adapting, and innovation-seeking activity.**

Relationships, Internal and External

The discussion thus far has dealt with the interrelationships among health administration programs, as compared to their external relationships. Environmental relationships relate to either *input constituencies*, those that supply resources of several kinds, or *output constituencies*, those that receive an organization's product. An organization may be rather *highly articulated and narrowly described* relative to these constituencies—of the nature of a closed system—or *poorly articulated and broadly described*, relative to these constituencies—of the nature of an open system. Further, an organization may be in relative *balance or imbalance* in respect to both sets of constituencies. Both of these circumstances are illustrated in Figure 2.

As in the case of relative concentration, the two main organizations in the educational field, AUPHA and ASPH, cannot be characterized in the same way relative to their several external constituencies. In general, it appears that AUPHA is an organization that has relatively

FIGURE 2

ORGANIZATION RELATIONSHIPS

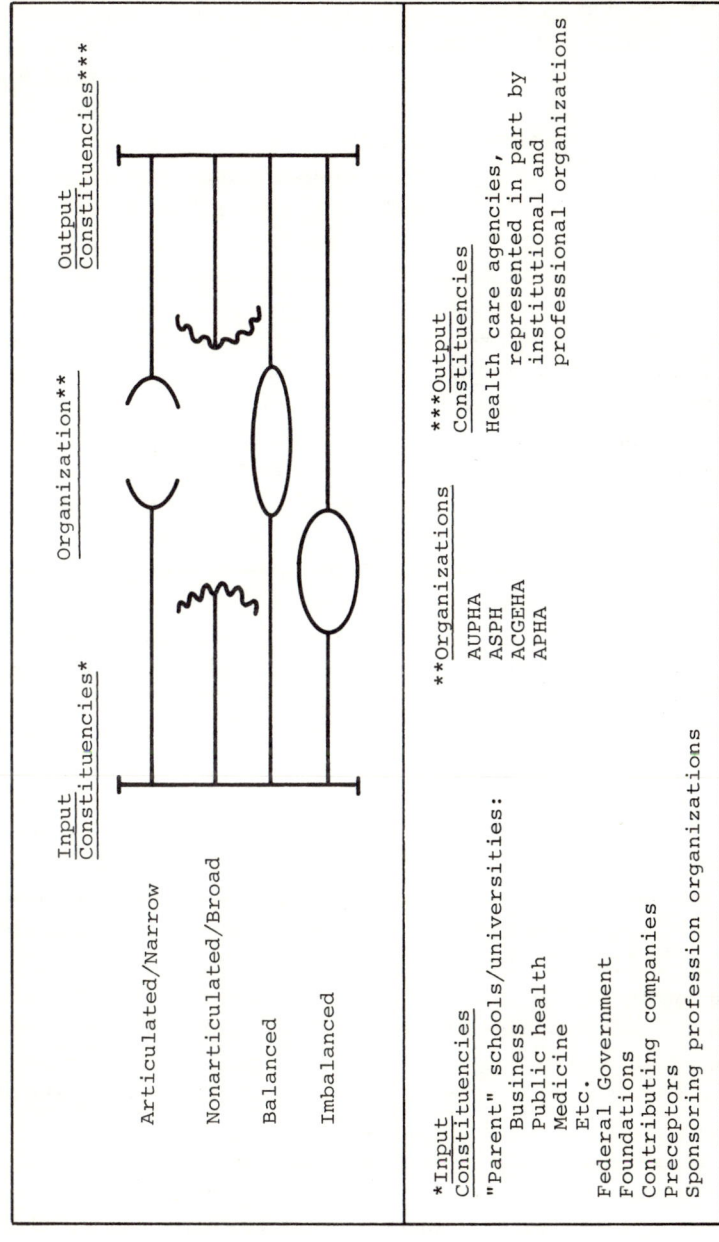

more diversified external relationships, both locally and nationally. On the input side, the relationships run strongly to occupational traffic, narrowly described in several instances to hospital administration. It appears that ASPH's relationships are less diversified, running strongly to the federal government and APHA at the national level.

Restated in terms of the organization/environment abstraction presented in Figure 2, AUPHA appears to possess fairly well-articulated relationships with numerous constituencies, but these relationships have not led to agreement on appropriate educational output; input relationships are over-balanced relative to output relationships. ASPH has strong relationships with one national constituency, i.e., articulated and delimited, with greater agreement on educational output, but less built-in capacity to consider alternatives.

The above attempt to classify and describe both organizational sets understates the real differences between them. Both operate with national structures that are small enough for informal contacts and individual personalities to strongly impact the formal situations. Further, the two are derivatives of professional streams and histories which are vastly different: health vs. medical care, community vs. institutions, public funding vs. private funding, etc. There is no sense in ignoring these differences, they are very real and lead to differing and conflicting world views and motivations.

Yet, it remains clear that there is strong need in all of U.S. health care for improved organization and administration, recognized in part by the creation of this Commission.

The Commission should underscore the importance of effective resolution of the organizational territories into a more effective whole and recommend ways of accomplishing it. In general, the problem runs less to the organizational link within the educational establishment(s) and more to externalities.

The scope of the national structure in the field should be both expanded and loosened. This means that AUPHA must be less concerned with strictly defined membership questions and more concerned with making it possible and specifically encouraging the affiliation of constituencies which would expand its scope. It should provide for and encourage individual memberships where faculty groups are not in a position or do not care to seek institutional membership and generally provide for constituency groups to participate in AUPHA affairs without being forced to disaffiliate from other groups. It should be noted that during the past two years AUPHA has moved in this direction, through both formal changes of its bylaws and informal discussions with numerous groups. This momentum needs and deserves further support and outside assistance.

In view of the pivotal role of AUPHA, the Commission should recommend that a new examination of its scope and structure be undertaken. The situation is quite similar to that of the AAMC in the mid-sixties, and what is needed is a Coggeshall-type study and report[2]—outside appraisal and recommendation by a competent and broadly accepted person or group, with action recommendations as to organization structure and other changes that would accomplish the broader leadership and forum aspects outlined above.

On the output side, the practicing community of health administration needs to be better represented in the network. There are loud complaints about educational output from interested and competent proffessionals. The importance of participants of various sorts in health administration education is obvious. In professional education, the viewpoint of the practitioner is essential.

There is need for substantial improvement in town-gown relations: the Commission should underscore this, and recommend means of accomplishing it. Such means must go beyond the traditional liaison committees between associations, cross-memberships on committees, etc.

A specific council should be created, and given both immediate and ongoing responsibilities. Further, its leadership should be accorded high standing in the governance of the health administration education organization which evolves. As Austin has stated, "the health and medical care industry is the most highly professional industry in our society."[3] Because of this, it is important for academic institutions in this field, and the associations which represent them, to stand firmly distinct from the professional community: the town-gown distinction is important. But, for the distinction to be functional and not disfunctional there should be a group specifically designed to provide coordination and communication between the two. In this way, the proper contributions to health administration education of both professional and academic elements can be maximized.

Functions of the Network

In the context of a structure which is now taken to be broadly inclusive of academic elements and strongly linked to external constituencies, it is appropriate to examine the third dimension of Figure 1: functions. Five functions are as follows:

Quality: Development of capable faculty, assistance to faculty in curricula and course development, support of independent accreditation, inservice education of faculty, etc.

Manpower development: Anticipation of needs and changes in health administration, recruitment of high quality students, coordination of different educational levels, continuing education, etc.

Communications: Providing a forum for exchange of information, and participation.

National policy development: Shaping policy and direction as regards health administration education, including funding and including research necessary to support such policy development.

Research: Development of support for and stimulation of research by faculties.

In respect to each of these five, several specific recommendations follow. Again, the intent here is not to deal with specific substantive issues but rather suggest organizational mechanisms through which such issues can be dealt with by the educational establishment. Consistent with Figure 1 each will be discussed in terms of: (1) the degree of organizational concentration; and (2) the kinds of constituency relationships necessary to approach the activity.

Quality Study Group: Academic Setting and Structure. Many of the comments received and discussed by the Commission have to do with the "industry structure" of health administration education: program size, relationships to other producers, vertical and horizontal integration, etc. Presumably, its recommendations will deal with these subjects.

As a follow up to the Commission's report, and because the issues require ongoing attention, AUPHA, probably in collaboration with ASPH and perhaps also with the American Assembly of Collegiate Schools of Business, should establish an ongoing study group on academic setting and structure. The group should include university officials and faculty other than health administration faculty, and should be asked to render reports periodically and no less than annually. The reports would be distributed to academic officials responsible for health administration offerings, association officials, accreditation groups, professional bodies, and others.

A partial list of subjects for such a group to address is as follows:

- Generalist vs. specialist education
- Appropriate size of graduate programs—minimum and maximum[4]

- Enhancing the strength and standing of health administration programs and faculty vis-a-vis their universities
- Single vs. multiple school sponsorship of programs
- Graduate/undergraduate education coordination
- Proper academic setting for health services research
- Proper setting for production of advanced degree scholars for teaching and research

A number of these topics are being addressed by the Commission, and the recommended study group would serve as a vehicle for further consideration and implementation. The field of health administration education is now at the stage where comparative analyses of some of these issues would be productive.

Manpower Development

A new council (or otherwise named group) reflecting town-gown interests has been recommended above. This group, contrary to the one proposed immediately above on academic structure, should be composed heavily of practicing professionals, and should have a voice in the governance of the revised AUPHA.

Part of this group's obligation would be to deal—again, in the manner of follow-up to recommendations of the Commission, and on an ongoing basis—with the following manpower questions:

Recruitment of high quality and qualifiable students.[5]—This is a legitimate concern of such a group because of the overlap in recruiting to *educational* programs and subsequent access to *professional* practices. Further, in a number of important cases—racial minorities and women—the impact of initial educational recruitment is strongly conditioned by subsequent acceptance and deployment of such persons in the practicing community.

Anticipation of manpower needs and changes. Aside from the supply and demand questions of numbers, there are the complicated questions of role definition.

Continuing education. The academic level of most continuing education in the field is atrocious, and the efforts of many groups offering continuing education are poorly coordinated. Further, many program facilities are not involved in continuing education efforts. In one way or another, credentialing in health administration will likely mandate continuing education. The role of the academic programs in this needs to be both sharpened and expanded, including the possibilities of coordination of the efforts of others, certification of courses, and drawing faculties more directly into specific continuing education offerings through national association.

Field education. The residency is an important portion of many curricula in health administration. It has been criticized as being pedantic, poorly reintegrated with the academic portion and insufficiently supervised.[6] The process by which residencies are selected by both faculties and students needs reexamination, as well as the role of preceptors and their relationship to academia. The content of field education needs examination in the light of role models identified and recommended by the Commission.

Management development. Organized executive development programs have been used in the business community for many years, but are rare in health adminstration.[7] Their relevance and usefulness seem obvious.[8]

COMMUNICATION

In general, there is already substantial communication among those faculties which are a part of AUPHA. The dangers of "over-communication" have already been mentioned.

New relationships should be established with five groups: health planning, mental health, long-term care, primary care, and teachers of community medicine in schools of medicine.[9] The last group is important because of the gradually increasing interest in medical schools in the organization and economics of health care.

The above five constituencies are noted because of their fairly obvious exclusion. Other groups which should become a part of expanded scope of AUPHA are already somewhat related, but inappropriately so to long run needs and potentials. The main group is the faculties of health services administration of schools of public health. This relationship is complicated by the presence of overlapping accreditation machineries.

Graduate/Undergraduate Programs

Despite efforts of AUPHA, there remain serious problems of coordination between undergraduate and graduate levels of education for health administration—to the disadvantage of applicants and students of both types, and the practicing community.

The Commission should underscore the need that a network of local or regional coordinating structures be developed and staffed, if necessary.

National Policy Development

Federal funding for education in health administration will likely continue in the future, and there are non-dollar aspects of national government and private decision-making upon which health administration educators need and deserve influence. This influence is now obtained in major part through Washington offices of AUPHA and ASPH. This approach has numerous advantages, and at least two risks. One is the tendency to seek funds from whatever sources seem available at a given time, without regard for long run implications. The other is for competition or conflict to develop between the two associations, both seeking financial support from one stream of funding.

A long-run strategy group should be formed, including persons of both academic association and representatives of related professional associations, to map out strategic pathways for national funding and policy development in health administration education.

Research

Many faculties in health administration conduct no organized research, to the detriment of both their own academic standing and the field.

The question of national funding for research should be addressed by the strategy group proposed immediately above.

The question of improved quantity and quality of health services research by universities should be addressed by the study group on academic setting and structure, decribed in the section above dealing with quality.

Summary

The present organization in health administration, AUPHA, is well-established and performing effectively on many fronts. Yet, it needs to be broadened to incorporate academic units that reflect the most inclusive view of health administration education. Further, new mechanisms are needed to link academic programs, acting collectively, to other constituencies, notably the practicing community.

Several new structures have been recommended. Their exact names have not been specified, but their general purposes, scopes and compositions have been presented. Clearly, they should not operate apart from the present network, but as important extensions and modifications of it. Precisely how that is done should be considered by organizational analysts.

One purpose of these several new groups is to provide for follow up on the Commission's recommendations. Without such, much of the

Commission's efforts will be lost. This points to a weakness in one-time, blue ribbon commissions: they stand apart from the regular structure for purposes of objectivity, but lose leverage. Conversely, it would seem desirable to build more powerful adaptation devices into the organizational fabric of the educational establishment. This becomes more difficult as a national association grows in size and complexity, yet more essential. A second purpose of these recommendations, then, is to increase the "dynamic tension" of the network, by suggesting mechanisms which would force the inclusion of new academic viewpoints, by confronting town-gown issues more directly, and by increasing activities of self-appraisal.

Notes

1. Minutes of Fifth Commission Meeting, Commission on Education for Health Administration, Oct. 12, 13, 1973. p. 10.
2. Lowell T. Coggeshall. *Planning for Medical Progress through Education.* Association of American Medical Colleges, 1965.
3. Charles J. Austin. "What is Health Administration?" Commission on Education for Health Administration, October, 1973. p. 3.
4. T. E. Chester. *Graduate Education for Hospital Administration in the United States: Trends.* American College of Hospital Administrators, 1969. p. 7. "There has perhaps been too much preoccupation with the problems of size, and the fear of depersonalization . . . Perhaps too little attention has been given to the disadvantages inherent in 'smallness,' which prevent specialization among teachers, and, perhaps even more critically, provide insufficient strength for urgently needed research."
5. In this connection, the efforts of AUPHA in recruitment of minority students is entirely commendable, and *the Commission should underscore the importance of continuing this type of effort.*
6. Chester. op. cit. pp. 13–16.
7. One good example: University of Michigan Hospital and Medical School.
8. For discussion, see R. H. Stimpson and S. J. Taylor. *Executive Development for Graduates of Master's Degree Programs in Hospital and Health Care Administration.* Proceedings of a Conference. Graduate Program in Hospital Administration, School of Public Health, Earl Warren Hall, University of California, Berkeley, California 94702, 1973.
9. AUPHA's present efforts as regards the first three of these should not be ignored; to the contrary, these efforts should be further supported.
10. As recommended generally by the "Millis Report." *The Graduate Education of Physicians.* American Medical Association, 1966. And the "Carnegie Report." *Higher Education and the Nation's Health.* Carnegie Commission on Higher Education, 1970. p. 47.

health administration press

M2240 School of Public Health
The University of Michigan
Ann Arbor, Michigan 48104
(313) 764-1380

Lewis E. Weeks, Ph.D.
Editor

The Press was founded in 1972 with the support of the W. K. Kellogg Foundation as a joint endeavor of the Association of University Programs in Health Administration and the Cooperative Information Center for Hospital Management Studies.

Editorial Board
Professor John R. Griffith
Chairman
University of Michigan

Avedis Donabedian, M.D.
University of Michigan

Gary L. Filerman, Ph.D.
Association of University
Programs in Health Administration

Professor Nora Piore
Columbia University

Lawrence D. Prybil, Ph.D.
Virginia Commonwealth University

David B. Starkweather, Dr.P.H.
University of California, Berkeley

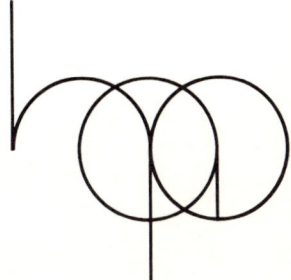

RA
440.6
C58
1975
v.2

SEP 1 1977